STONEWELL

HEALING PRESS

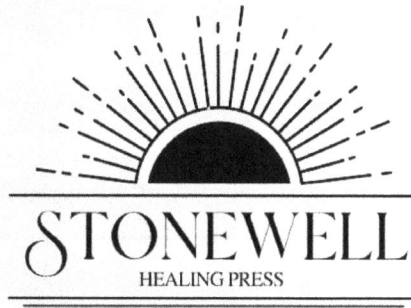

Thank you for being here. We're honored to walk beside you.

M. Tourangeau

Stonewell Healing Press

TABLE OF CONTENTS

Stonewell Healing Press

TABLE OF CONTENTS

Stonewell Healing Press

Dedicated to those who's heart
broke over drops of milk.

STONEWELL HEALING PRESS

HOW TO USE THIS WORKBOOK

Take your time with this. The more you pause to really think about each question and answer honestly, the more space you create for reflection. And with deeper reflection, this experience can open up new understanding and healing you might not expect.

Be honest with yourself—there's no judgment here. This is your private space. If you want, you can even throw this book away or burn it later to keep your secrets safe. That said, be mindful of how much you dive in. Healing and reflection around tough, sensitive topics can bring up strong feelings—and yes, it can get triggering. So here's your gentle trigger warning.

The real progress comes when you practice the skills, not just read about them. The more you try them out in your life, the more helpful this workbook will be.

ASSESSMENT

Before we begin, take a moment to honestly check in with yourself by rating these statements on a scale from 1 (not at all) to 10 (completely):

1-10

1. How connected do you feel to your baby during feeding or caregiving moments?

2. How much guilt or self-blame do you carry related to your feeding experience?

3. How comfortable are you acknowledging and expressing anger, frustration, or grief about your feeding journey?

4. How supported do you feel — by medical providers, family, or your community — in your feeding experience?

5. How well do you trust your body and its ability to care for your baby?

6. How able are you to soothe or calm your nervous system when you feel overwhelmed or triggered by feeding challenges?

7. How free do you feel from cultural or familial pressure or judgment regarding your feeding choices?

8. How confident are you in your capacity to heal emotionally from your breastfeeding experience?

SECTION ONE

The Myth of Natural and Easy — What You Were Told vs. What Actually Happened

You were told this would be natural. That your body would know. That it would be simple — maybe a little uncomfortable at first — but deeply bonding, intuitive, and beautiful. And so, when it wasn't, you didn't just struggle... you questioned everything. Your instincts. Your body. Your worth. And worst of all, your love.

You're not alone.

What no one tells you is how violent it can feel to be blindsided by something that was supposed to be "instinct." You weren't broken — you were unprepared for a reality no one warned you about. You were grieving something you didn't even know you had expectations for. That grief is real. That shame is real. And that story deserves to be rewritten with the truth: you did not fail. You were told a story that didn't leave room for your humanity. This chapter begins the work of gently dismantling that lie.

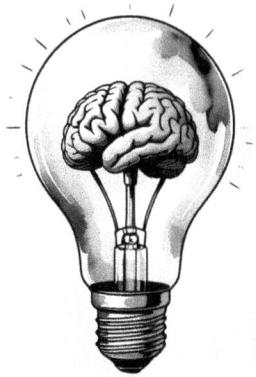

Making Sense Of It
Breaking the "Perfect Mother" Trap

The belief that breastfeeding should come naturally is one of the most persistent myths of motherhood — and it's a myth that's quietly reinforced everywhere we look. From social media to parenting books to casual conversations with well-meaning friends and family, the message is the same: if it isn't flowing smoothly, if it isn't effortless, something must be wrong with you. Subtle cognitive distortions creep in: "I should be able to do this perfectly," "Other mothers seem to manage just fine," "If I struggle, I'm failing." These "should" statements build invisible chains, linking your worth as a parent to an arbitrary standard of maternal perfection.

This pressure is not new. Across cultures and centuries, women's bodies have been scrutinized, judged, and commodified when it comes to feeding children. Wet nurses, formula debates, public breastfeeding taboos — all of these reflect a recurring cultural story: mothers are always accountable, always measured, and rarely allowed room to simply be. Modern "breast is best" campaigns, while well-intentioned, often echo this old message, turning what should be personal choice into yet another source of guilt, comparison, and anxiety.

When breastfeeding doesn't go as planned, it often triggers something deeper than disappointment. It touches the invisible tapestries woven during our own childhoods — early experiences that shaped how we see ourselves when we fail, when we are not enough, or when love and approval feel conditional.

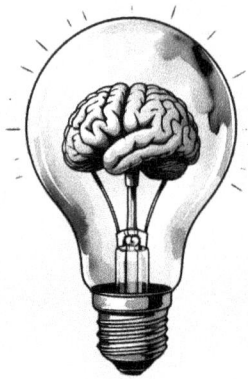

Making Sense Of It
Breaking the "Perfect Mother" Trap

"If I can't do it perfectly, I must be failing" is often the first whisper of a wound that predates motherhood. For many, breastfeeding difficulties reactivate old abandonment fears, shame from past mistakes, or narratives that measure self-worth against achievement. Suddenly, a struggle with milk supply or latching isn't just practical — it becomes a judgment on your very identity.

The internal dialogue can become relentless. Thoughts like:

- "If I loved my baby enough, I would have made it work."
- "Something is wrong with me — other women can do it."
- "I failed my child before I even got started."

These are not truths; they are echoes of societal expectations, perfectionism, and trauma. They feel urgent and absolute, but they are distortions — stories that your inner critic has learned to repeat, often louder than your own inner voice of compassion.

The impact is real. Mothers may feel isolated, anxious, or profoundly inadequate. They may mourn a version of motherhood that never existed or judge themselves harshly for struggles that are biologically, socially, and emotionally normal. And yet, when we step back, the larger truth emerges: breastfeeding is deeply personal, variable, and influenced by countless factors beyond effort or love. By examining these distorted beliefs and the cultural pressures that feed them, mothers can begin to disentangle identity from performance.

What were you told — directly or indirectly — about what breastfeeding should be like?

Take your time to gently recall the messages you absorbed from family, books, nurses, online forums, or culture. These might not have been explicit — sometimes it's what wasn't said that carries the most pressure. Try not to censor yourself. This isn't about blame — it's about awareness.

What were you told — directly or indirectly — about what breastfeeding should be like?

How did your actual experience differ from the story you were sold?

Let yourself speak freely here. Where did things become confusing, painful, or disorienting? What emotions came up when reality clashed with expectation? This is a space for your anger, your disappointment, your heartbreak. It's safe to name it.

How did your actual experience differ from the story you were
sold?

What did you start believing about yourself when feeding became hard?

Go inward. When things weren't working, what stories formed about you — your body, your worth, your adequacy as a mother? Did old wounds around failure, abandonment, or rejection come up? What did your inner child believe in those moments?

What did you start believing about yourself when feeding became
hard?

Were there moments you felt judged — even silently — by others?

Explore how the presence or silence of others shaped your experience. Did a comment from a nurse, a glance from a friend, or a scroll through social media deepen your shame? Name those moments without self-censorship.

Were there moments you felt judged — even silently — by others?

Who would you be — or how would you feel — if this story didn't mean anything about your worth?

Let yourself imagine: what if this feeding experience wasn't a measure of your love, your value, or your future as a mother? Who would you be without the shame? Let this prompt stretch you toward freedom.

Who would you be — or how would you feel — if this story didn't mean anything about your worth?

What do you wish someone had said to you in the hardest moments?

Write it now — as if speaking to yourself. Let it be warm, wise, and full of the empathy you needed then. This can become part of your healing language.

What do you wish someone had said to you in the hardest
moments?

TRACING THE TRUTH

REFLECTING ON CULTURAL MESSAGES

From social media posts to advice from family or healthcare providers, mothers are constantly bombarded with messages about how feeding "should" happen. This exercise helps you separate external pressures from your own authentic experience, so you can define what success truly means for you and your baby.

Why it helps:
By identifying which messages are borrowed and which align with your values, you reclaim agency over your feeding journey. This reflection reduces shame, clarifies your own priorities, and supports self-compassion in the face of cultural expectations.

List the Messages You've Received
- Write down everything you've heard about breastfeeding from society, family, friends, media, and healthcare providers.

Separate Truth from Expectation
- Ask yourself: "Which of these messages feel true for me? Which are borrowed expectations?"

Redefine Success
- **Write a paragraph describing what success in feeding** looks like for you personally — beyond judgment, comparison, or societal standards.

TRACING THE TRUTH

REFLECTING ON CULTURAL MESSAGES

Messages You've Received	Does this feel true to me?

Redefine Success

TRACING THE TRUTH

REWRITE THE TRUTH

Cultural messages and internalized "shoulds" can make breastfeeding feel like a test of your worth. This exercise helps you identify the myths you've absorbed and replace them with compassionate, realistic truths that honor both you and your baby.

Why it helps:
Naming the myths gives them power over you, while rewriting them allows you to reclaim your perspective. This shifts the focus from judgment and shame to self-compassion and clarity, helping you parent from a grounded, empowered place.

List the Myths You Believed
- Write down statements you felt you "should" follow about breastfeeding.
- Examples:
    - "Breastfeeding is what makes you a real mother."
    - "If you love your baby, it will come naturally."
    - "If it's hard, you're doing it wrong."

Write a Counter-Truth for Each
- Create compassionate, realistic statements that reflect your own experience and values.
- Examples:
    - "Being a real mother is about showing up with love — not about how milk is delivered."
    - "Sometimes, love means continuing even when it's hard. Sometimes, it means choosing a different path."

TRACING THE TRUTH

REWRITE THE TRUTH

Myths You Believed	Counter-Truth

TRACING THE TRUTH

LETTER TO YOUR HOPES

Breastfeeding often doesn't go as we imagined, and the gap between expectation and reality can stir grief, shame, or frustration. Writing a letter to the feeding experience you hoped for gives you a safe place to express those feelings, honor your effort, and cultivate self-compassion.

Why it helps:
This exercise helps you release shame, process grief, and separate your worth from cultural expectations or imagined ideals. By putting your feelings into words, you create space for healing and self-acceptance.

Write Your Letter
- **Begin with:** "Dear Feeding I Imagined" or "Dear Dream I Had"
- **Describe what you hoped the breastfeeding experience** would feel like.
- **Write honestly** about what actually happened and how it made you feel.

End with a self-affirmation, for example:
"I was always a good mother — even when this was hard."
Read it aloud if it feels safe, then take a few deep breaths.

TRACING THE TRUTH

LETTER TO YOUR HOPES

TRACING THE TRUTH

LETTER TO YOUR HOPES

TRACING THE TRUTH

LETTER TO YOUR HOPES

TRACING THE TRUTH

LETTER TO YOUR HOPES

MASK WORK

We all carry layers — the parts we show and the parts we protect. Trauma, stress, or social expectation often make us overinvest in the "front" mask while ignoring the care the "back" side needs. This exercise gives you a safe way to explore both sides without forcing exposure. By naming what's hidden, you acknowledge your needs; by sharing a small sliver with a trusted person, you practice vulnerability and connection without danger. It helps build trust in yourself — that you can both protect and reveal, and that your inner life is valid and worthy of care. Over time, you may notice your outer mask feels lighter, more authentic, because your inner self has space to be seen.

Fill Them In — List words, phrases, or images for each side. Don't censor yourself.

Choose a Safe Reveal — Pick one tiny sliver from the Back mask and plan to share it with a safe person this week.

Reflect — Notice what it feels like to acknowledge and/or reveal that part of yourself.

What the world sees　　　　　　　　**What you protect or that needs care**

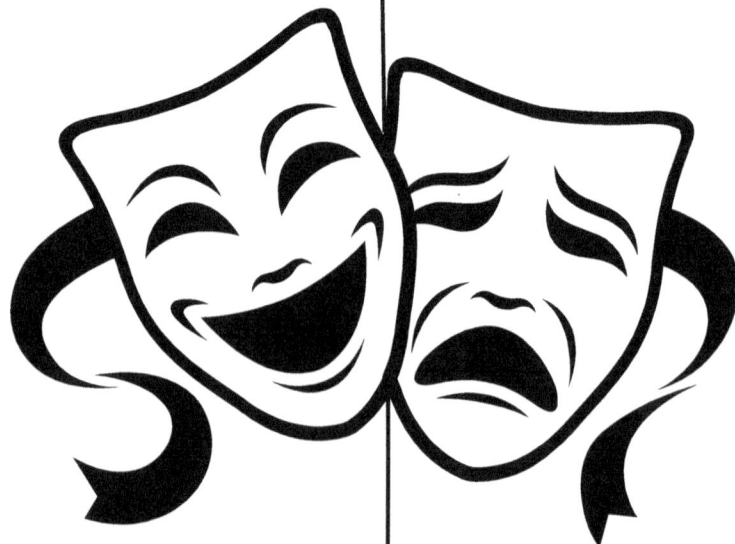

FEELING IN MOTION

Our bodies carry what words often can't — tension, joy, grief, or relief. Moving intentionally helps you process and release emotions stored in the body, while giving a tangible sense of your day's narrative. Ending in a posture of strength signals to your nervous system: I survived, I'm here, I can hold myself steady. This isn't about dancing perfectly or performing for anyone; it's about giving your inner experience a voice through movement, noticing how small gestures can express complex feelings. Over time, this practice reconnects body and mind, helping you feel grounded, seen, and resilient.

Choose a Song — Something that matches or invites movement for your current state.

Move Freely — Let your body express today's story. Small gestures count — a hand to heart, a sway, a shrug.

Notice — Pay attention to tension, ease, or areas that want attention.

End in Strength — Finish in a posture that conveys groundedness and safety (feet planted, shoulders relaxed, chest open). Hold for 30 seconds.

Reflect — Journal a few words about what your body expressed and how it feels afterward.

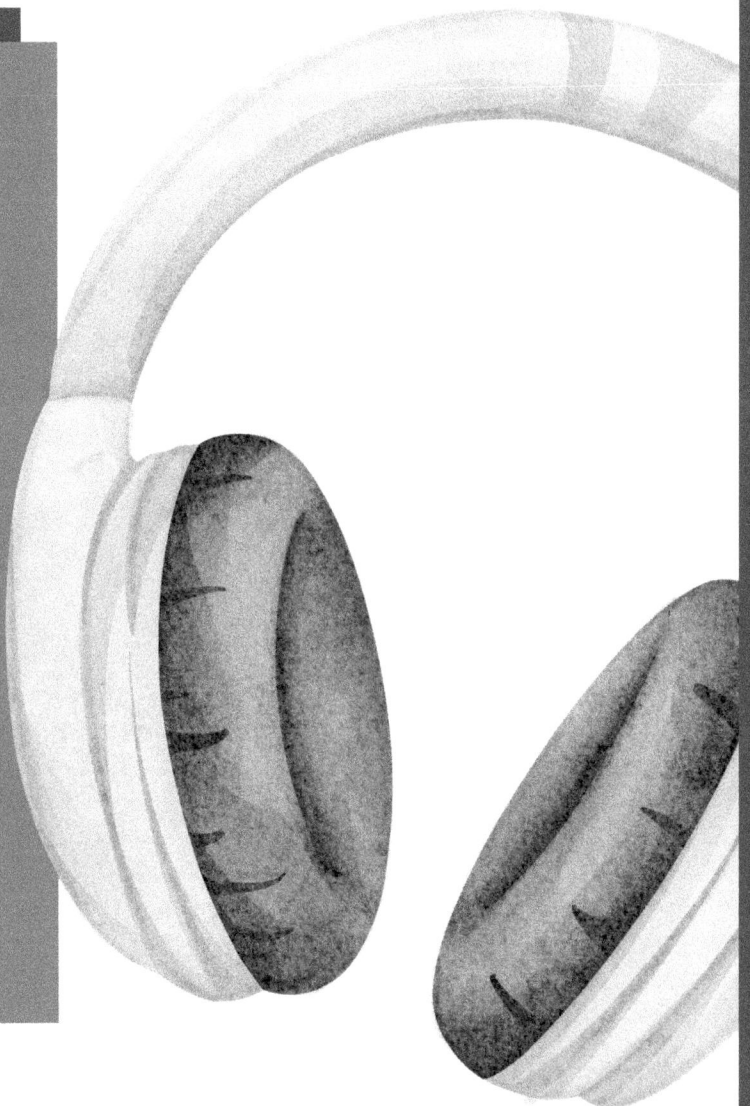

SECTION TWO

When It Starts Before It Starts — Birth Trauma, NICU, and Medical Complications

For many mothers, the trauma of breastfeeding doesn't begin at the breast. It begins on a hospital bed, in an ambulance, under surgical lights, or beside a plastic incubator where your baby was taken — too soon, too fast, without you. It begins when the plan unravelled before your arms ever held your child.

Maybe you couldn't hold them right away. Maybe there were wires, beeping monitors, rushed nurses. Maybe you were numb, stitched, stunned. Maybe you were bleeding, shaking, alone. Whatever happened, it matters — because that rupture becomes the soil breastfeeding tries to grow in.
And when it doesn't go smoothly, it's not your fault.

The feeding journey was shaped before it ever began.
This chapter is about telling the truth of what you survived — and giving yourself the grace you were never offered. What you carried was never "just birth." It was trauma. And that trauma has a right to be seen.

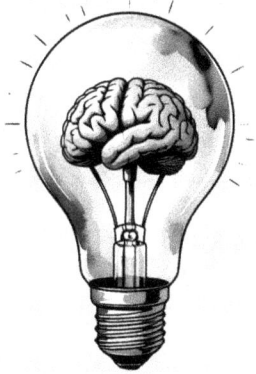

Making Sense Of It

How Early Trauma Shapes the Feeding Journey

Even before your first latch, the body remembers. The moments immediately after birth — the separation, the interventions, the shock — create a subtle blueprint for how you experience feeding, touch, and maternal connection. When your baby was whisked away, or when your body felt violated, out of control, or unsafe, those memories can embed themselves in the nervous system. Later, when breastfeeding feels challenging, your mind and body may respond not just to milk supply or latch issues, but to echoes of fear, loss, and helplessness from those first hours.

Culturally, we are taught that breastfeeding should be "natural" and seamless, but anthropology tells a different story: across societies, infant feeding has always been a negotiated, embodied practice — rarely perfect, often communal, and always influenced by stress, trauma, and environment. Mothers have fed under duress, illness, or social constraints, and the pressure to perform "perfectly" is a modern invention. When our birth experiences were traumatic, that cultural pressure compounds the difficulty, layering shame and self-blame over already vulnerable emotions.

Early trauma can create internalized narratives like:
- "My body failed me before I even tried."
- "If this doesn't work, I'm failing as a mother."
- "I should feel joy and connection, but I don't."

These are not truths. They are survival patterns: your nervous system learned to protect you in moments of threat.

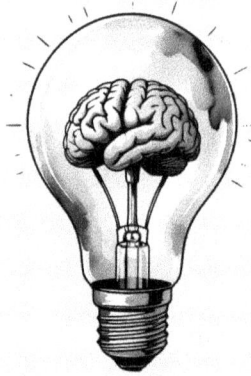

Making Sense Of It

How Early Trauma Shapes the Feeding Journey

Your body may interpret difficulty as danger because it associates feeding with the moments of fear or loss from birth. Recognizing this reframes the struggle: the challenge is not evidence of inadequacy, but a normal response to abnormal circumstances.

Healing begins with acknowledgment. When we name the trauma, validate its impact, and give ourselves permission to mourn the moments that were stolen, we reclaim the foundation for connection. Breastfeeding difficulties are rarely about willpower; they are about safety, regulation, and compassion — for yourself and your baby. By witnessing what you endured, understanding its influence, and offering yourself grace, you can begin to untangle early trauma from current experience, creating space for healing, trust, and embodied maternal confidence.

Even small gestures — a gentle touch, a pause before a feeding, a moment of eye contact — can begin to rewrite the nervous system's memory of threat. Trauma doesn't have to dictate the future of your feeding relationship. By creating moments of safety, attuning to your body's signals, and giving yourself permission to let go of expectations, you gradually teach both your body and mind that nourishment can be experienced with presence, connection, and care. This is not about "fixing" anything; it's about reclaiming agency over your body, your rhythm, and the way you bond with your child, one mindful, compassionate step at a time.

What happened during your birth, and how did it affect your ability to feed?

This doesn't need to be clinical or detailed unless you want it to be. Just tell the truth in your own words. What emotions or sensations do you still carry from those early hours? Did you feel seen, rushed, supported, or dismissed?

What happened during your birth, and how did it affect your ability to feed?

Were there moments you felt separated — physically or emotionally — from your baby?

Whether it was NICU, a delayed first hold, surgical recovery, or simply shock and disconnection, name those moments. What impact did that separation have on how you felt as a mother?

Were there moments you felt separated — physically or emotionally
— from your baby?

What kind of support did you need after birth — and what did you actually receive?

Were you pressured to perform? Left alone with feeding expectations? Rushed into choices your body or heart weren't ready for? Write without filtering. This is your truth, not your apology.

What kind of support did you need after birth — and what did you actually receive?

Did your body feel like it belonged to you during the early postpartum period?

Explore your relationship with your body after birth. Did you feel invaded, touched without consent, out of control? What did you need in order to feel safe in your own skin again?

Did your body feel like it belonged to you during the early postpartum period?

Have you ever connected the dots between your birth story and your breastfeeding struggle?

Let this be a gentle exploration — not to create blame, but to offer context. When feeding is difficult after a traumatic start, it makes sense. Let your nervous system feel that logic.

Have you ever connected the dots between your birth story and your breastfeeding struggle?

What does your body still remember — even if your mind has moved on?

Use this as an invitation to check in with your physical self. Any tightness? Numbness? Grief stored in your chest, throat, or belly? Your body may hold pieces of the story that your mind has tried to minimize.

What does your body still remember — even if your mind has moved on?

TRACING THE TRUTH

FEEDING TIMELINE REFLECTION

Every feeding session carries the weight of both past experiences and present reality. Looking at your feeding journey as a timeline allows you to see progress, patterns, and moments of resilience — without judgment.

Why it helps:
This exercise helps you notice triggers, celebrate small wins, and separate current challenges from earlier trauma. It builds awareness and self-compassion by giving structure to a process that often feels chaotic.

Create a timeline: Draw a simple line across a page. Mark the birth date at the start.

Plot significant feeding moments: Include both challenges and positive experiences — latching issues, pumping sessions, bonding moments, or relief.

Reflect on patterns: Note any recurring triggers or moments of ease.

Add self-compassion notes: For each difficult moment, write a short compassionate statement, e.g., "I did my best under difficult circumstances."

TRACING THE TRUTH

FEEDING TIMELINE
REFLECTION

TRACING THE TRUTH

FEEDING TIMELINE
REFLECTION

MOOD MAPPING BY THE HOUR

Our mood is never random — it's deeply influenced by what we do, when we do it, and how our nervous system responds. When depression or anxiety is heavy, it can feel like nothing makes a difference. This log helps you prove to yourself that even small activities shift your emotional state, sometimes by just one point. And that one-point lift matters — it's momentum, a reminder that you aren't stuck forever. By tracking your mood alongside your activities, you build a personalized map of what nourishes you. Instead of relying on guesswork, you'll have hard evidence of your own resilience patterns. Over time, this practice shows you that certain choices (a call with a safe friend, a walk outside, finishing a task) consistently bring relief. This isn't about forcing happiness — it's about noticing what gently nudges you toward better.

For one day, each hour, write down what you're doing and your mood (0–10).

Repeat for a few days — notice patterns.

Circle activities that reliably lift you by at least one point.

Intentionally schedule more of those "one-point lifts" into your week.

Revisit the log whenever you feel stuck, to remind yourself you have options.

Day	Activity	Mood Before	Mood After

MOOD MAPPING BY THE HOUR

Day	Activity	Mood Before	Mood After

SELF-COMPASSION BREAK

When stress, shame, or pain flare up, most of us go straight into self-criticism: Why can't I handle this better? What's wrong with me? That inner attack only tightens the spiral. Kristin Neff's Self-Compassion Break interrupts that cycle. It gives you three small handholds: recognition of your pain, the reminder you're not alone in it, and an active choice to soften instead of harden against yourself. With repetition, your nervous system learns that you don't have to white-knuckle through suffering or numb out — you can meet yourself with the same tenderness you'd extend to a friend. That shift doesn't erase the pain, but it changes the way it lands in your body. Over time, it builds resilience, because you're no longer abandoned in hard moments; you become your own safe ally.

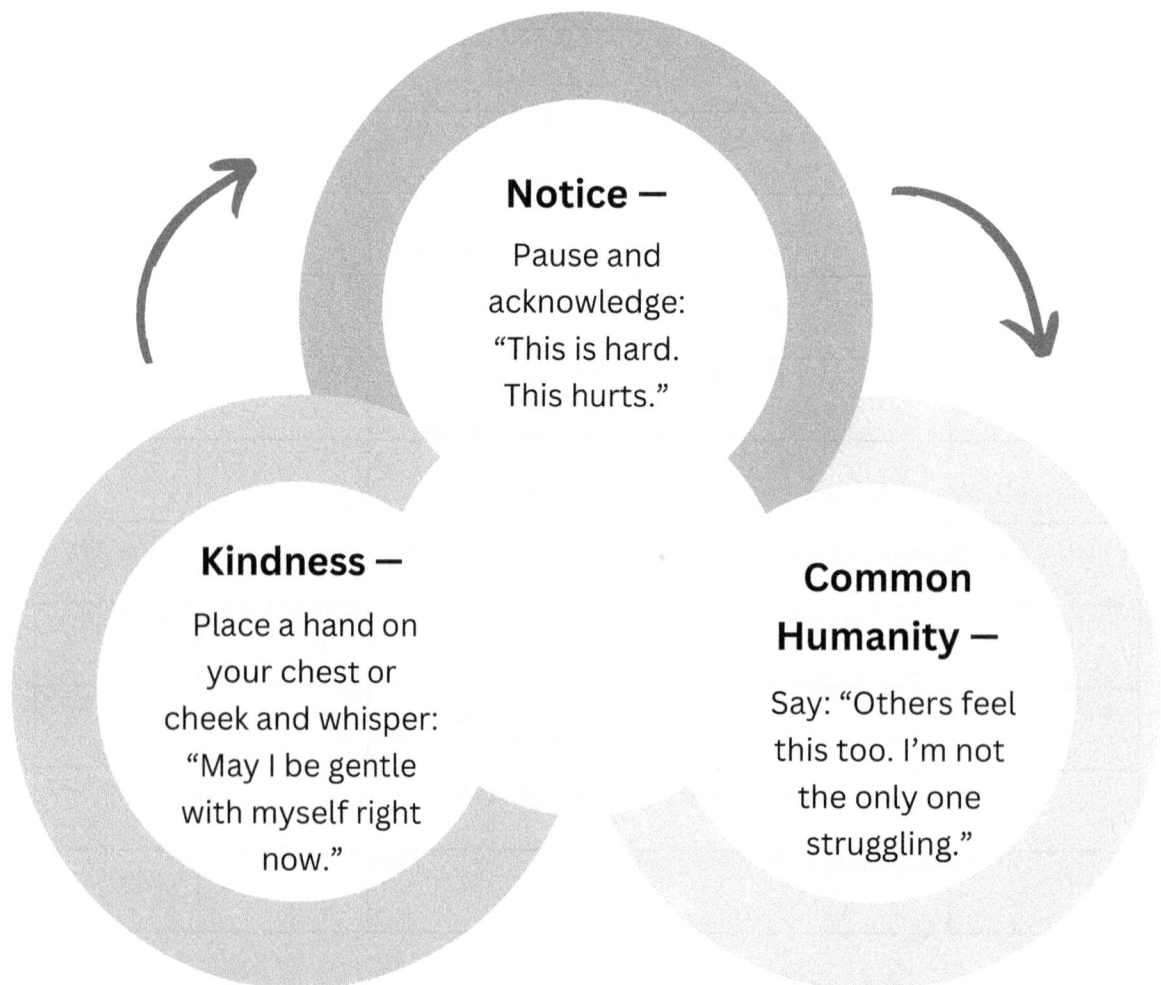

Notice —
Pause and acknowledge: "This is hard. This hurts."

Kindness —
Place a hand on your chest or cheek and whisper: "May I be gentle with myself right now."

Common Humanity —
Say: "Others feel this too. I'm not the only one struggling."

POCKET MOOD LIFTERS

When life feels heavy, it's easy to forget what actually helps. In hard moments, the brain tends to focus on what's wrong, not what's available. An Antidote List is your preloaded reminder: ten small, proven things that shift your state even a little. These aren't grand fixes or instant cures — they're micro-adjustments that keep you from sliding deeper into the stuckness. Pairing an antidote before a hard task helps you face it with steadier energy; using one after provides recovery and closure so you don't carry the weight forward. Over time, this list becomes muscle memory — your nervous system learns, When I struggle, I have options. That's the opposite of hopelessness.

1 **List Ten** — Write down 10 things that reliably lift your mood (a song, a walk, fresh air, texting a safe friend, lighting a candle). Keep them small and doable.

....

....

....

....

....

....

....

....

2 **Use Before** — Pick one before facing a task you tend to dread. Let it soften resistance.

3 **Use After** — Choose another as a closing ritual. Let it tell your body, That part is done. I'm safe again.

SECTION THREE

Not Enough of Anything — Sleep, Milk, Help, Time, or Support

You were running on empty. Not metaphorically — literally. No sleep. No silence. No real help. You were asked to feed a baby every two to three hours, around the clock, while your body bled, your hormones crashed, and your mind stretched thin with fear and pressure.

And if milk didn't come easily — or at all — the panic set in. Maybe you pumped for hours. Maybe you tried every supplement. Maybe your baby screamed at the breast and you screamed into a pillow. Maybe you whispered, "I'm trying. I'm trying." But no one seemed to hear it.

This chapter is about honoring the reality of maternal depletion — the deep, invisible cost of doing too much with too little for too long. You didn't fail. You were failed by a culture that expects you to give endlessly without rest, nourishment, or meaningful support. It's time to tell the truth about what it took — and what it took from you.

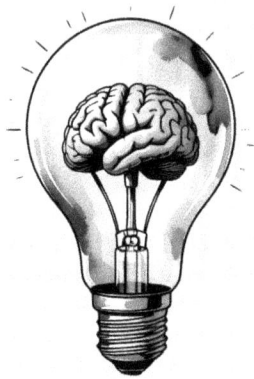

Making Sense Of It

The Invisible Cost of Maternal Depletion

The postpartum period is often framed in books, media, and cultural narratives as tender, joyful, and "magical." In reality, for many mothers, it is relentless, exhausting, and isolating. You are expected to love endlessly, give constantly, and respond immediately — all while your body is recovering from birth, your hormones are fluctuating wildly, and your nervous system is still learning how to regulate after trauma. Anthropologists note that in most traditional human societies, newborn care was never a solo task. Mothers were supported by extended family, neighbors, and communal networks. The modern mother, however, often faces the opposite: cultural glorification of self-sacrifice paired with minimal support. The result is maternal depletion that goes unseen, under-acknowledged, and misunderstood.

Sleep deprivation alone reshapes perception, memory, and emotional regulation. Chronic lack of sleep floods the nervous system with stress hormones, leaving mothers more reactive, more anxious, and more likely to internalize self-blame. When this interacts with breastfeeding challenges — painful latching, low supply, frequent pumping, or inconsolable crying — guilt and shame become nearly unavoidable. Mothers report believing, "If I loved my baby enough, I could fix this," or "Other mothers manage this, so something is wrong with me." These messages are not truths; they are the echo of a society that equates maternal worth with capacity for endurance and emotional labor, rather than realistic support and self-care.

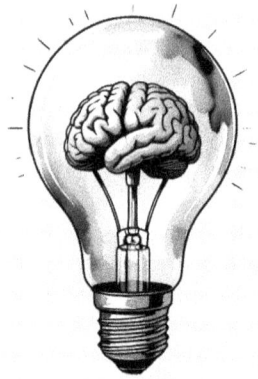

Making Sense Of It
The Invisible Cost of Maternal Depletion

Feeding itself becomes a physical and emotional battleground. Every attempt, every session, carries the pressure of doing it "right." You may have measured ounces, timed sessions, or tried every supplement, all while your body begged for rest, nourishment, and touch. Your nervous system is wired to survive, not perform perfectly; functional freeze, dissociation, and emotional numbness are normal responses to prolonged stress. Yet when mothers experience these states, they often interpret them as moral or personal failure, not as survival mechanisms designed to protect themselves and their babies under extreme conditions.

Culturally, the expectation that a mother should give endlessly is reinforced by family, healthcare, media, and social norms. Social media amplifies this pressure, presenting curated images of "effortless" breastfeeding, smiling mothers, and content babies. It can feel as though everyone else is succeeding while you are floundering — but these portrayals are illusions, not reality. Real feeding journeys are messy, challenging, and profoundly human. Understanding that the "perfection myth" is cultural, not personal, is essential to breaking cycles of self-blame.

The psychological impact of maternal depletion is profound. Chronic under-support affects self-esteem, confidence in parenting, and attachment experiences. Mothers may feel isolated in their struggles, thinking, "I'm alone in this," when, in truth, this experience is shared by many, though rarely acknowledged.

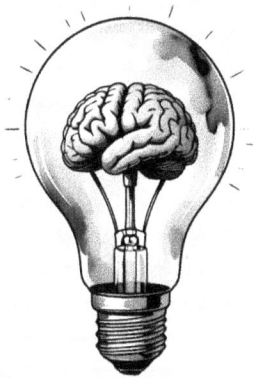

Making Sense Of It
The Invisible Cost of Maternal Depletion

Emotional and somatic awareness — noticing where exhaustion, tension, or anxiety live in the body — is a vital tool for regaining agency. DBT strategies, radical validation, and gentle reflection create space to recognize the truth: You were doing the job of an entire village, alone.

Healing begins with acknowledgment. Naming the depletion, grief, frustration, and anger validates your experience. Recognizing the structural and cultural pressures that set the stage for exhaustion externalizes blame, freeing you to offer yourself compassion. When you see the invisible labor for what it was — monumental, courageous, and exhausting — shame begins to lose its power. Recovery is not about "fixing" yourself; it is about reclaiming your body, your time, your emotional bandwidth, and your trust in your instincts.

By witnessing the true cost of maternal depletion, you reclaim not only compassion for yourself but also a more grounded relationship with your baby. Boundaries, realistic expectations, and self-care are not indulgences; they are necessities. Feeding is not a moral test, and your worth is not measured by supply, endurance, or uninterrupted care. This insight reframes the narrative from guilt and shame to truth, survival, and the beginning of restoration. The invisible cost is finally named, and with that acknowledgment comes the first steps toward healing, empowerment, and gentler, more sustainable motherhood.

What did you need more of — but didn't get — in those early weeks?

Sleep, time, kindness, food, space to cry, someone to say "you're allowed to rest." What were you desperately craving but couldn't name? Let yourself grieve the absence of what should have been provided.

What did you need more of — but didn't get — in those early weeks?

What were you told you "should" be able to do — and how did that pressure shape your experience?

Explore the hidden expectations: "Breastfeed exclusively," "Nap when the baby naps," "Just relax and it will work." What was expected of you that felt impossible? What did that do to your sense of worth?

What were you told you "should" be able to do — and how did that pressure shape your experience?

What strategies did you use to keep going when you were running on fumes?

Sometimes we dissociate. Sometimes we go into overdrive. Sometimes we collapse. What did you do to survive the impossible? Reflect with compassion — survival is not weakness, it's brilliance.

What strategies did you use to keep going when you were running on fumes?

How did the feeding experience interact with your sleep deprivation or emotional state?

Feeding every two hours, setting alarms to pump, dreading the next latch — how did this affect your ability to rest or recover? Did you start to fear the nights? Did you begin to lose parts of yourself?

How did the feeding experience interact with your sleep
deprivation or emotional state?

Who do you wish had stepped up — and what would support have looked like?

Name names, if it helps. Partner, family, providers, friends. Be honest. Not to blame, but to acknowledge the vacuum. What kind of care did you need?

Who do you wish had stepped up — and what would support have looked like?

If someone else told you this same story, how would you respond to them?

Let yourself answer with the empathy you rarely give yourself.
What would you say to a friend who had lived what you lived?

If someone else told you this same story, how would you respond to them?

TRACING THE TRUTH

SELF-VALIDATION LETTERS

When exhaustion and guilt are constant companions, giving yourself permission to acknowledge the truth of your experience is essential. Writing a letter to yourself allows you to honor both your effort and your limits.

Why it helps:
This exercise reinforces self-compassion, shifts the narrative from shame to truth, and strengthens your internal support system during challenging feeding periods.

Find a quiet, safe space and take three grounding breaths.
Write a letter to yourself starting with: "Dear Exhausted, Doing-Too-Much Me"
Include the following points:
Acknowledge what you endured: sleepless nights, endless feeding, emotional labor.
Validate your love and effort: "Even when I was exhausted, I showed up."
Offer compassion and permission to rest: "It's okay to need help and it's okay to pause."

Read aloud or keep private, revisiting whenever guilt or self-blame arises.

TRACING THE TRUTH

SELF-VALIDATION LETTERS

TRACING THE TRUTH

SELF-VALIDATION LETTERS

TRACING THE TRUTH

MICRO-BREAK MAPPING

Even small moments of rest matter. In a period defined by sleep deprivation and constant care, identifying opportunities for micro-breaks can reduce chronic stress and support nervous system regulation.

Why it helps:
Recognizing and using even brief pauses interrupts the cycle of depletion, helping you regulate emotions, reduce guilt, and reconnect with your body.

Mark feeding sessions, sleep, and self-care moments from a typical day. Identify micro-break opportunities — 2–5 minutes of deep breathing, sipping water, stretching, or simply closing your eyes.

Commit to one micro-break per feeding cycle for the next week. Write a note about how it made you feel physically and emotionally.

TRACING THE TRUTH

MICRO-BREAK MAPPING

06:00	
07:00	
08:00	
09:00	
10:00	
11:00	
12:00	
13:00	
14:00	
15:00	
16:00	
17:00	
18:00	
19:00	
20:00	
21:00	
22:00	
23:00	
24:00	

TRACING THE TRUTH

THE INVISIBLE LOAD INVENTORY

Motherhood often involves countless invisible tasks — mental, emotional, and physical — that pile up without acknowledgment. This exercise helps you name and honor the weight you carried, from feeding to emotional labor, so you can see your effort clearly and validate your experience.

Why it helps:
Putting your "invisible load" on paper externalizes it, reducing overwhelm and shame. It highlights how much you were doing and helps you see where support is needed.

List everything you were responsible for during the early postpartum and feeding period. Include feeding-related tasks, worry, planning, pumping, sleep interruptions, and household tasks.
Reflect on your effort: Next to each item, write a brief acknowledgment: e.g., "I did this under extreme exhaustion; I survived."

Optional: Highlight tasks that could have been shared or delegated — this helps envision support structures for the future.

TRACING THE TRUTH

THE INVISIBLE LOAD INVENTORY

Mental Load	Emotional Load	Physical Load

TRACING THE TRUTH

THE INVISIBLE LOAD
INVENTORY

Mental Load   **Emotional Load**   **Physical Load**

SHELF IT FOR LATER

Sometimes intrusive images or thoughts crash in like uninvited guests — too loud, too vivid, too much. Trying to "not think about it" only makes them louder. Containment gives your mind a safe boundary. Instead of battling the thoughts, you acknowledge them, then choose to store them somewhere secure until you're resourced enough to revisit them (ideally with therapeutic support). This isn't avoidance — it's wise pacing. By practicing containment, you send a message to your nervous system that you're in charge of when and how you engage. It builds trust with yourself, lowers overwhelm, and allows you to get through the present moment without drowning in unfinished business.

Visualize a container
Pick something sturdy — a jar, vault, chest, box, or even a digital safe.

Name the intrusion
Briefly identify the image, memory, or thought you want to contain. Write it in this jar here.

Place it inside
Imagine physically setting it in the container.

Seal it shut
Hear the latch click, see the lock turn, or feel the heaviness of the lid close.

Store it away
Place the container on a high shelf, deep cave, or secure room in your mind.

Return only with support
Remind yourself you can revisit it later with a therapist, journal, or trusted guide.

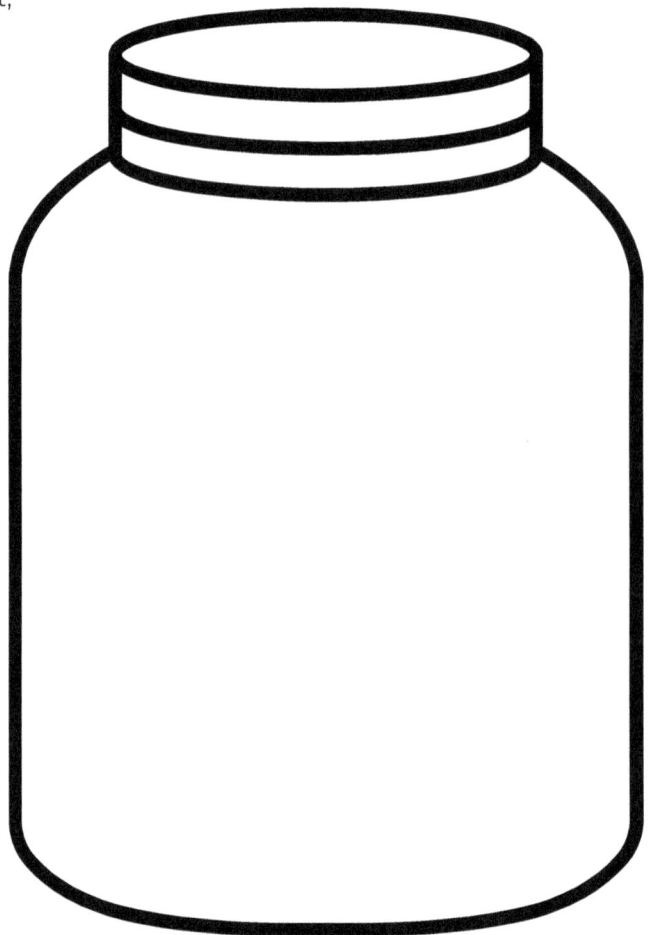

LESSONS IN INK

After hardship, the brain often circles around the why — why it happened, why you stayed, why you're still hurting. Meaning-making is a way to gently reclaim authorship. By naming what you survived and drawing out what it taught you about your own values and limits, you shift from being swallowed by the story to becoming the narrator of it. This process isn't about silver linings or forced positivity. It's about grounding your pain in context — saying, this mattered, this shaped me, and here's what I'm carrying forward. Closing with a boundary sets a line in the sand: you're not just reflecting on what happened, you're deciding how it changes the way you'll protect yourself in the future.

Headline: Write a short, bold line that sums up what you survived (as if it were on the front page of your personal newspaper).

Lessons: List 3–5 things it revealed about your needs, your limits, or your values.

Boundary: Write one clear, non-negotiable boundary you'll honor from now on.

SECTION FOUR

When Care Wasn't Care — Medical Harm, Dismissal, and Systemic Failure

You reached out for help. You asked the questions. You trusted the experts. You followed instructions, even when it didn't feel right. You did everything "they" said. And still — it hurt. It didn't work. Or it worked at a devastating cost.

For so many, breastfeeding trauma is not just about what went wrong — it's about how no one seemed to care that it did. When care is rushed, dismissive, contradictory, or coercive, it doesn't just leave you unsupported. It leaves you injured. Whether it was the nurse who yanked your baby's head to your breast, the lactation consultant who said "just push through the pain," or the doctor who made you feel hysterical — you were harmed.

And still, you may have blamed yourself.
This section helps you name what happened. Because bad care is trauma. And healing requires seeing that what was done to you — or neglected entirely — was never your fault.

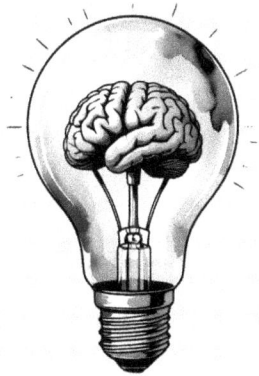

Navigating Systemic Gaps and Professional Limits

Many mothers approach breastfeeding with hope, determination, and trust. They reach out to lactation consultants, pediatricians, family doctors, and nurses, expecting guidance, clarity, and support. Yet too often, the care they receive falls short — not because of a lack of effort, but because the system itself is fragmented, under-resourced, and inconsistent. Family doctors, while well-intentioned, frequently lack sufficient training in lactation science, leaving mothers with advice that feels vague, contradictory, or outright unhelpful. Even IBCLCs may be varied in skill level, and are limited in availability, constrained by appointments, or bound by institutional protocols. The result is a landscape where even the "best care" may not meet your needs, answer your questions, or honor your lived experience.

For many, this creates a painful paradox: you do everything "right" — you follow guidance, track feeds, try supplements, attend appointments — and yet the struggles persist. The emotional fallout can be significant. Mothers often internalize the messages they hear, thinking, "If it's not working, it must be me" or "I'm failing my baby". These beliefs are reinforced by cultural myths that breastfeeding should come naturally, that professionals always know best, and that mothers should quietly persevere. The truth is that the limitations are systemic and structural, not personal. Breastfeeding is a biological, emotional, and social process shaped by many variables — infant temperament, maternal physiology, prior trauma, sleep deprivation, and support systems. Even highly trained professionals can only do so much.

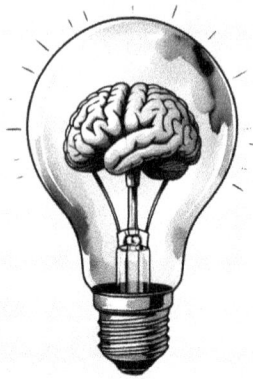

Making Sense Of It

Navigating Systemic Gaps and Professional Limits

Miscommunication, rushed consultations, or incomplete guidance does not mean your effort is insufficient or that your bond is compromised. Trauma often emerges not only from physical difficulties but from being dismissed, unheard, or invalidated at a moment of extreme vulnerability. Feeling hurt by inadequate care is not shameful — it is human.

This section invites you to name the gaps in care, the missed opportunities for understanding, and the frustration of trying to navigate conflicting advice. Radical validation is key: your questions, concerns, and emotional responses are legitimate. You are allowed to mourn the support you did not receive, recognize the limits of even skilled professionals, and honor your perseverance despite systemic failure. Recognizing these truths helps disentangle self-blame from external failure, rebuild trust in your instincts, and create a framework for self-compassion in the ongoing feeding journey.

Healing here is not about "perfect care" or recreating an ideal experience. It is about acknowledging the reality: care sometimes fails, knowledge is imperfect, and support is uneven. Naming this truth allows you to give yourself the compassion you were rarely given, reclaim your agency, and recognize that seeking help — and persevering — in an imperfect system is itself an act of courage and resilience.

What did "professional help" look or feel like in your experience?

Was it warm and supportive? Cold and clinical? Contradictory or rushed? Try to name not just the facts, but how your nervous system responded. Did you feel safe? Seen?

What did "professional help" look or feel like in your experience?

Were there moments you felt dismissed, gaslit, or pressured by someone you trusted to help you?

This might be hard to admit — especially if you were taught not to question authority. Write what happened. Write what you couldn't say then.

Were there moments you felt dismissed, gaslit, or pressured by someone you trusted to help you?

Did any part of your body or intuition protest, even silently, during those interactions?

This is where your inner wisdom lives. Reflect on what your body felt or wanted to say, even if you didn't speak it out loud. That truth still matters.

Did any part of your body or intuition protest, even silently, during those interactions?

What parts of you tried to stay "good" or compliant during these experiences?

Were you afraid of being labeled dramatic, difficult, or noncompliant? Did you freeze or fawn? Give voice to the parts of you that tried to stay safe.

What parts of you tried to stay "good" or compliant during these experiences?

What did you need from your providers or support team — and what was missing?

Was it softness? Permission? Patience? Clarity? Consistency? Make a list, not to create blame — but to validate what you were starved for.

What did you need from your providers or support team — and what was missing?

Have you blamed yourself for things that were the result of poor or harmful care?

Gently name the moments where self-blame crept in. Ask yourself: Was this truly my failure — or the result of someone else's negligence or pressure?

Have you blamed yourself for things that were the result of poor or harmful care?

TRACING THE TRUTH

Not all care is equal, and not all professionals have the knowledge or resources to support you fully. Reflecting on your experiences with medical staff, IBCLCs, and doctors can help you separate personal responsibility from systemic failure.

Why it helps:
This exercise validates your struggle, identifies where support failed, and helps release unnecessary self-blame.

List every professional you consulted during your feeding journey.
Next to each, note what guidance or support you received.
Identify gaps, contradictions, or moments you felt dismissed or unheard.
Write a short compassionate statement to yourself: "I did my best within the limits of the system. Their failure is not my failure."

TRACING THE TRUTH

THE PROFESSIONAL CARE REFLECTION

Professionals You Consulted

Guidance Received

Gaps & Contradictions

Compassionate Statement to Yourself:

TRACING THE TRUTH

CONFLICTING ADVICE JOURNAL

Breastfeeding often involves navigating contradictory advice from multiple sources, which can leave you confused and doubting yourself. Documenting these experiences helps you see patterns and reclaim clarity.

Why it helps:
This exercise externalizes the confusion, validates your decision-making process, and strengthens trust in your instincts.

Write down every conflicting piece of advice you received about feeding, latch, or supply.
Note how each piece made you feel — stressed, guilty, frustrated, or anxious.
Reflect on the advice you ultimately followed and why.

End with a statement affirming your choices: "I made the best decision I could with the information I had. I trusted my instincts."

TRACING THE TRUTH

CONFLICTING ADVICE JOURNAL

Advice

Feelings

Your Choice

Affirmation In Your Choice

Advice

Feelings

Your Choice

Affirmation In Your Choice

TRACING THE TRUTH

CONFLICTING ADVICE JOURNAL

Advice

Feelings

Your Choice

Affirmation In Your Choice

Advice

Feelings

Your Choice

Affirmation In Your Choice

SAFETY IN SENSATION

After stress, trauma, or relational upheaval, our bodies often feel like a battleground—tense, guarded, or disconnected. Reclaiming the body is about coming back home to yourself. By practicing gentle, nurturing touch, you signal to your nervous system that it's safe to soften. This isn't indulgence; it's essential care. Daily attention to your physical self strengthens body awareness, lowers chronic tension, and reminds you that your body is a safe place, not just a vessel for pain. Over time, these small acts become proof: I can care for myself, and my body can be trusted again.

1 **PICK A NURTURING TOUCH**
Examples include rubbing lotion into your hands, sinking into a warm bath, wearing soft or comforting clothes, or even a gentle hand on your chest.

2 **ENGAGE FULLY**
Notice textures, warmth, weight, or scents — bring mindful awareness to the sensation.

3 **BREATHE INTO THE TOUCH**
Let each inhale gather calm, each exhale release tension.

4 **PRACTICE DAILY**
Even 2–5 minutes consistently signals safety and care.

5 **NOTICE CHANGES**
Check in with your body and note any softening, release, or increased comfort over time.

WORRY WINDOW

Worries often hijack your mind, showing up at every unexpected moment. By giving them a dedicated "time slot," you reclaim control instead of letting them run your day. This practice teaches your nervous system that there's a safe space and a safe time to process, so you're not constantly reacting to every intrusive thought. During the window, you can gently evaluate what's actionable versus what you need to let go, building clarity and self-trust. Outside the window, a simple cue like "not now—later" helps you return to the present without guilt or shame. Over time, this simple structure reduces the intensity and frequency of anxious loops.

Park your worries: Write them down as they arise.

....

....

....

....

Set a 15-minute window: Choose a consistent time each day for processing.

....

Outside the window: Use a cue phrase like "not now—later" to return to your day.

Inside the window: Review the list. Solve what's actionable, accept what isn't, and release judgment.

Close the window: End with a grounding or soothing activity to signal completion.

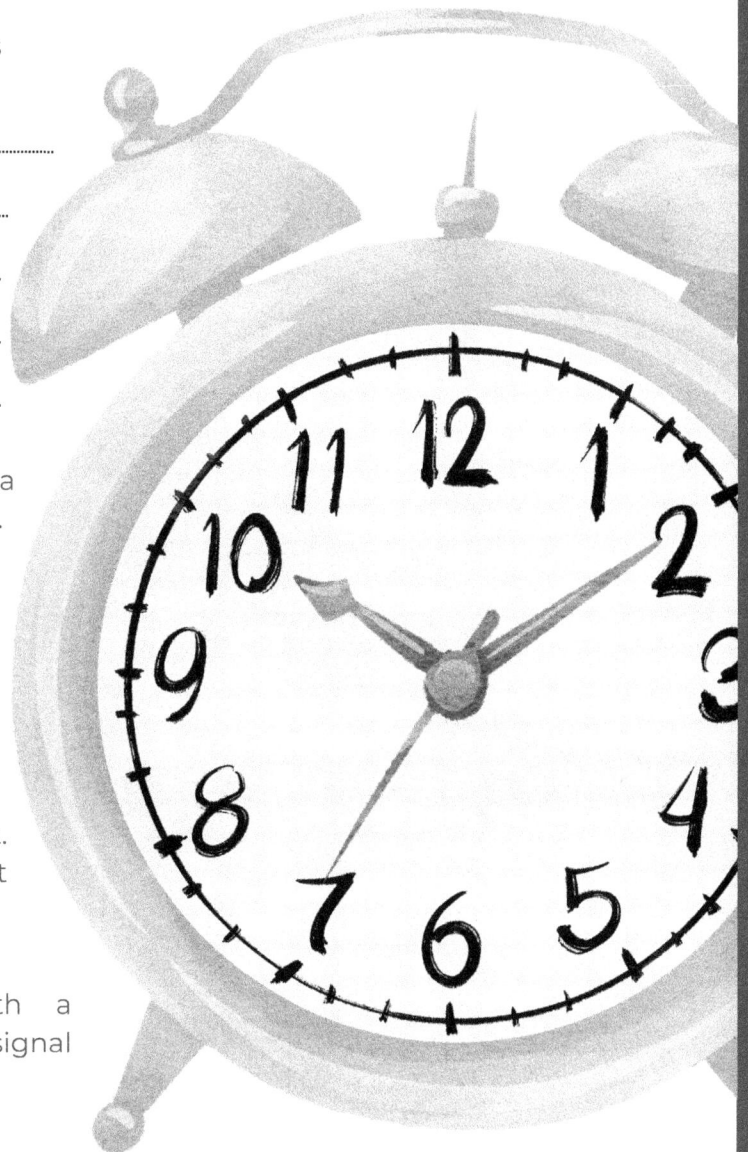

SECTION FIVE

The Body in Pain — Bleeding, Mastitis, Touch Aversion, and Physical Trauma

Your body wasn't just tired — it was torn, raw, aching, inflamed. Maybe your nipples bled. Maybe mastitis took you down with fever and chills. Maybe you winced at every latch or recoiled when someone touched your chest. Maybe no one told you how painful it could be.

Breastfeeding is so often romanticized — soft-focus images of serene mothers and sleepy babies. But for many, it was brutal. And when the pain is dismissed, invalidated, or minimized, it becomes more than physical — it becomes traumatic.

You might still feel a flinch when your baby cries, not because you didn't love them, but because your body remembers the agony. You may carry silent shame for resenting your baby or feeling disconnected during those painful moments. This section is here to say: you are not weak, broken, or ungrateful. You were in pain. And your pain deserves to be acknowledged, unraveled, and released — not minimized or endured in silence.

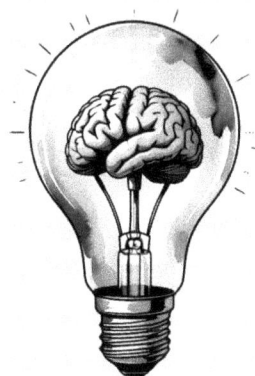

Making Sense Of It
When Physical Pain Becomes Trauma

The body is memory. Every twinge, every flare of pain, every involuntary flinch is the nervous system's way of saying, "I survived this." For mothers who experienced bleeding, mastitis, painful latches, or touch aversion during breastfeeding, the physical experience is inseparable from the emotional and psychological impact. Trauma is not defined solely by dramatic events; it is often measured by the body's response to prolonged, repetitive stress — and breastfeeding pain can fall squarely into this category.

Culturally, motherhood is glorified as effortless, intuitive, and tender. Western media saturates us with images of serene mothers cradling calm babies, seamlessly feeding on cue. For those whose experiences were agonizing, this ideal creates a profound cognitive dissonance: "If breastfeeding is supposed to feel natural, why does my body scream 'no'?" The result is shame, guilt, and a disconnection from both body and baby. Mothers may internalize thoughts like, "I shouldn't hate this moment" or "I must be doing something wrong," when in reality, the body is simply protecting itself from pain.

From a physiological perspective, repeated pain signals trigger the nervous system to enter a state of hypervigilance. The body learns to anticipate injury, creating flinches, muscle tension, or withdrawal — even when the threat is gone. Mastitis, nipple trauma, and other complications amplify this feedback loop, reinforcing fear, stress, and anxiety around feeding. Add in exhaustion, hormonal shifts, and societal pressure, and you have a perfect storm where physical pain becomes enmeshed with emotional trauma.

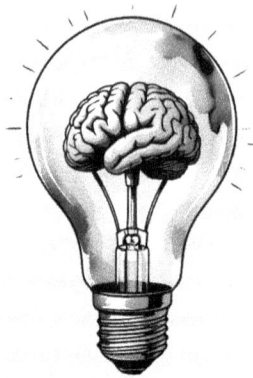

Making Sense Of It
When Physical Pain Becomes Trauma

Emotionally, this creates a duality: deep love for your child alongside a visceral, protective aversion to the source of pain. This is normal. Feeling resentment, irritation, or disconnection in the moment does not make you a bad parent — it makes you human. Trauma-informed care emphasizes that acknowledging pain, rather than minimizing or pushing through it, is essential for healing. The goal is not perfection or endurance; it is recognition, understanding, and compassionate integration of body and mind.

DBT and somatic awareness offer tools to disentangle trauma from ongoing care. Recognizing bodily responses as communication rather than failure allows mothers to engage with feeding in ways that honor both their baby's needs and their own limits. Naming the physical reality, processing emotional responses, and reclaiming agency over touch and proximity fosters healing — a gradual rebuilding of trust between body, mind, and infant. Your body remembers what your mind sometimes cannot fully articulate, and giving that memory acknowledgment is not optional; it is vital.

In this section, you are invited to witness your physical pain with radical compassion, disentangle it from guilt or shame, and learn that the body's protective signals are valid. By naming, exploring, and understanding the intersection of physical trauma and maternal identity, you reclaim authority over your body, reconnect with your infant without fear, and begin to release the lingering weight of pain that was never meant to be carried in silence.

What physical pain did you experience while breastfeeding — and how would you describe it, in your own words?

Go beyond clinical language. Describe the felt sense: Was it burning? Searing? Electric? Constant or throbbing? Giving your pain language honors its reality.

What physical pain did you experience while breastfeeding — and
how would you describe it, in your own words?

How did others respond to your pain — and how did that shape your own story about it?

Did they say "That's normal"? Did they brush it off? Or treat you like you were being dramatic? Let yourself feel what those dismissals cost you.

How did others respond to your pain — and how did that shape
your own story about it?

Were there moments when you dreaded your baby's cry — not because you didn't love them, but because you knew what was coming?

This is a tender one. If so, write about it with zero judgment. You were not heartless. You were hurting.

Were there moments when you dreaded your baby's cry — not
because you didn't love them, but because you knew what was
coming?

Did you ever feel like your body betrayed you — or like you couldn't trust it?

Explore what stories you started telling yourself about your body during and after this experience. Let your body respond, too.

Did you ever feel like your body betrayed you — or like you couldn't trust it?

What did you need your body to hear from you then — and what does it need now?

Imagine holding your body the way you would a wounded friend. What do you want to say to it now, with compassion?

What did you need your body to hear from you then — and what does it need now?

Have you been able to feel safe in your body since then — or has some part of you stayed tense, guarded, or shut down?

Name where the tension still lives. You don't need to fix it right now — just witness it.

Have you been able to feel safe in your body since then — or has some part of you stayed tense, guarded, or shut down?

GENTLE BREATH FOCUS

When anxiety spikes, the mind and body race together — thoughts accelerate, heart rate climbs, muscles tighten. Counting your breath gives both something steady to follow. By pairing inhale and exhale with numbers, you create a gentle anchor that slows the nervous system, refocuses attention, and interrupts spiraling thoughts. This isn't about perfection or achieving ten — it's about returning to the rhythm whenever distraction occurs. Even a few minutes daily strengthens your capacity to notice tension, settle your body, and move through anxious moments with less overwhelm.

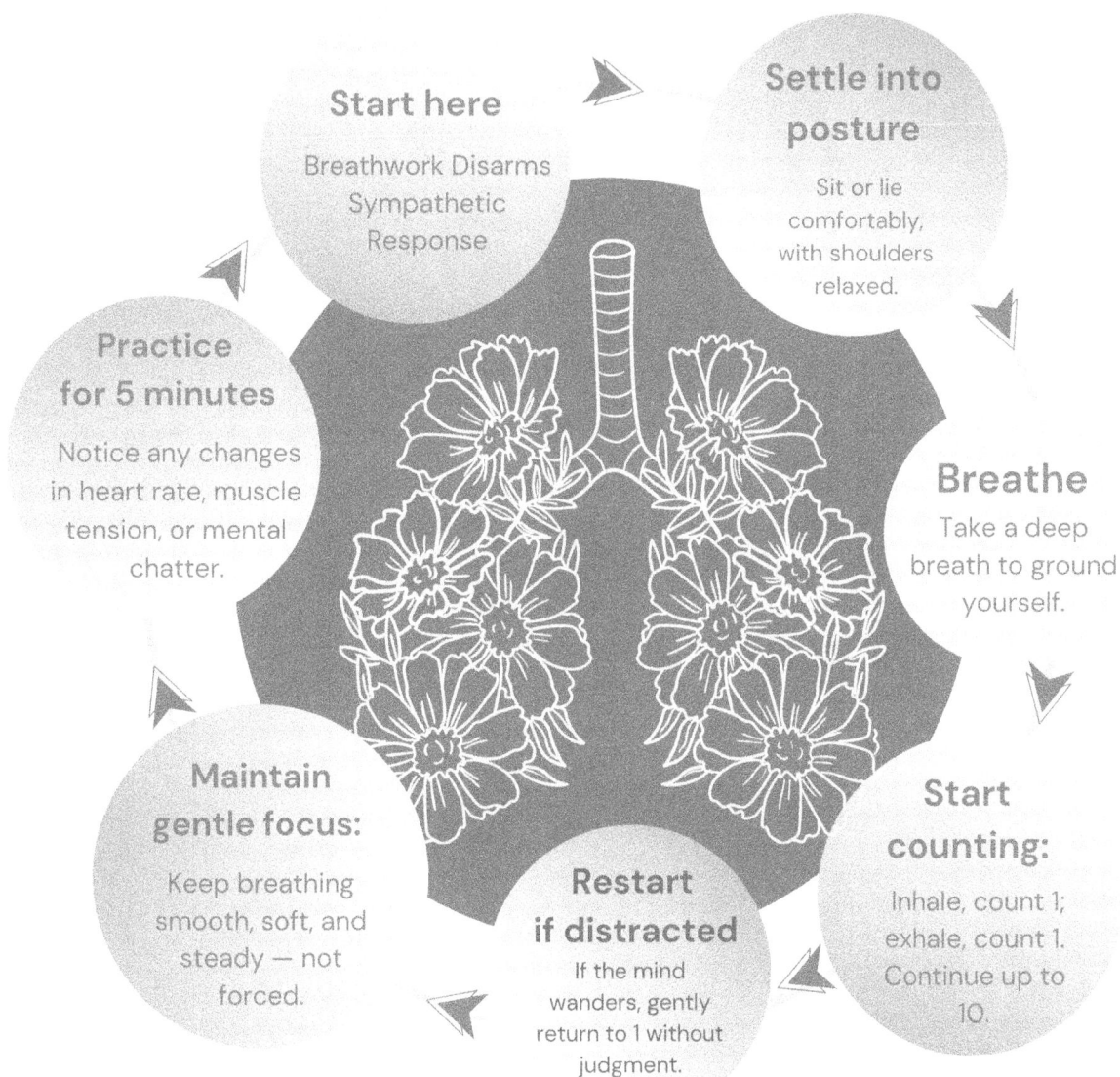

Start here
Breathwork Disarms Sympathetic Response

Settle into posture
Sit or lie comfortably, with shoulders relaxed.

Breathe
Take a deep breath to ground yourself.

Start counting:
Inhale, count 1; exhale, count 1. Continue up to 10.

Restart if distracted
If the mind wanders, gently return to 1 without judgment.

Maintain gentle focus:
Keep breathing smooth, soft, and steady — not forced.

Practice for 5 minutes
Notice any changes in heart rate, muscle tension, or mental chatter.

TRACING THE TRUTH

PAIN MAPPING

Your body carries memory. Mapping where you felt pain during feeding helps externalize it, acknowledge it, and reduce its emotional intensity.

Why it helps:
Labeling and visualizing pain validates your experience and begins to separate your body's trauma from self-blame.

On the next page, use to the body outline and mark areas where you experienced pain — bleeding, mastitis, latch-related soreness, or tension. **Next to each mark, write how the pain felt emotionally** (fear, dread, frustration).

Reflect briefly: "My pain was real. My body was communicating its needs. I did not fail."

TRACING THE TRUTH

PAIN MAPPING

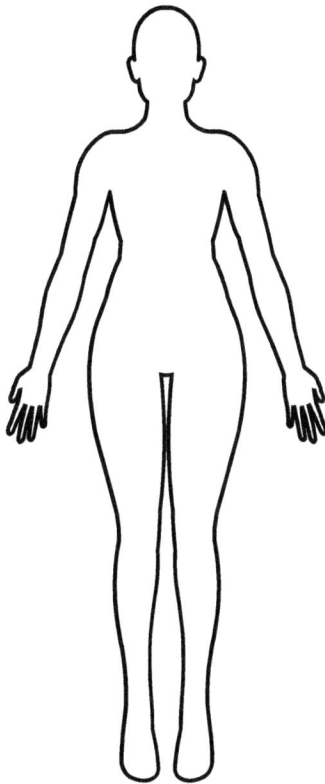

PROGRESSIVE MUSCLE RELAXATION

When stress lingers, tension builds in muscles without us noticing, keeping the nervous system on high alert. PMR gently signals to your body that it's safe to let go. By intentionally tensing and then releasing each muscle group, you highlight the difference between tension and relaxation, training your body to notice and release stress. This practice doesn't just relax the muscles—it communicates to your nervous system that it can downshift, making calm feel real and accessible.

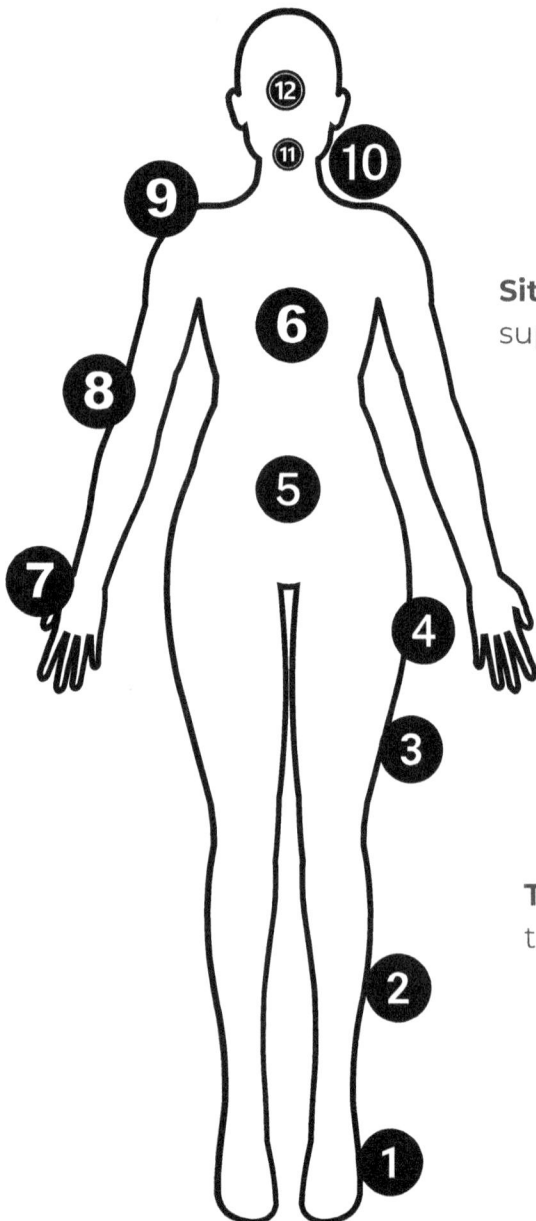

Sit or lie comfortably with your body supported.

Starting at your feet, tense the muscles for 3–5 seconds, then exhale and release.

Move upward through calves, thighs, glutes, stomach, back, hands, arms, shoulders, neck, jaw, face, tensing and releasing each group.

As you release, imagine tension melting away or flowing out of your body.

Take a few normal breaths and notice the overall sense of ease.

THE VOO RESET

Our vagus nerve connects the brain and body, regulating stress and calm. Gentle vocalization, like a long "voo" on the exhale, stimulates this pathway, sending a signal that it's safe to downshift arousal. The vibration through your chest and throat also grounds your attention in your body, giving your nervous system tangible proof that it can relax. Just a few rounds can reduce tension, slow your heart rate, and invite a sense of ease.

Sit or stand comfortably with shoulders relaxed.

Inhale slowly through your nose.

Exhale while vocalizing a long, gentle "voo," letting your chest and throat vibrate.

Repeat for 3 rounds, noticing the sensations and any shift in tension.

Place a hand on your chest to feel the vibration more clearly.

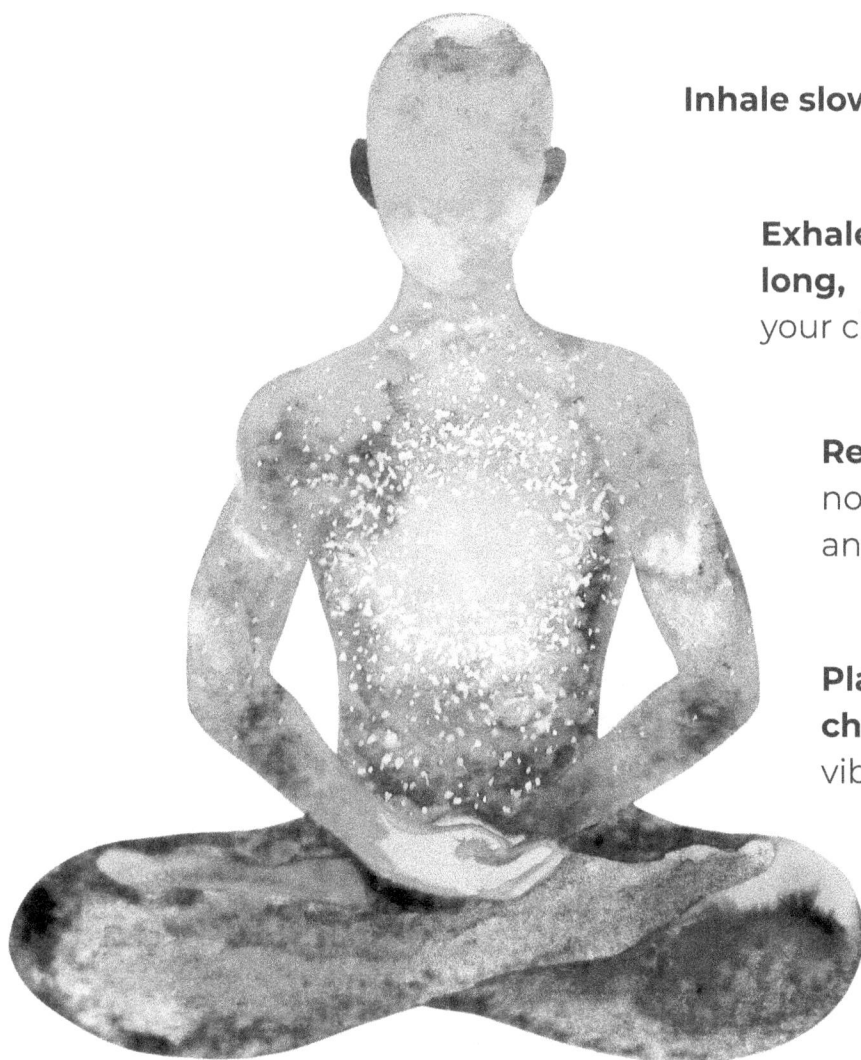

SECTION SIX

Cultural and Family Pressure — When Everyone Had an Opinion but No One Held You

Maybe your mother said, "We all did it — you'll be fine."
Maybe strangers stared as you reached for a bottle.
Maybe you were told, directly or silently, that "real mothers breastfeed."

Cultural myths and family expectations have a way of curling around your choices like vines — choking your voice, erasing your experience, piling shame on top of struggle. When breastfeeding became hard — or impossible — maybe you felt like everyone had something to say... but no one actually asked how you were.

This section is a soft place to lay down the weight of judgment — and name what you endured. You're not broken for feeling angry, resentful, or defensive. You were cornered by expectation. You were told to sacrifice, smile, perform — while suffering in silence. You don't owe anyone an explanation. You don't have to convince anyone that your pain was real. But you deserve to understand the full impact of what happened — and let it go.

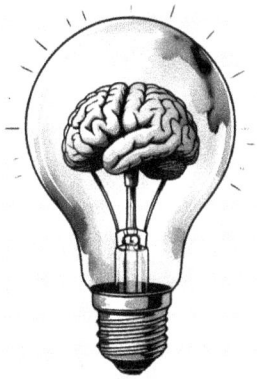

Making Sense Of It

The Weight of Expectation and Silent Judgment

Motherhood does not happen in isolation. From the moment a baby arrives, the world has opinions, rules, and standards — many of them unspoken. Family members, friends, and even strangers may weigh in, offering advice, critique, or judgment, often under the guise of "help" or tradition. Cultural myths about breastfeeding — that it should be natural, easy, and defining of "good mothering" — are reinforced across generations, social media, and even professional spaces. These messages can wrap around a mother like invisible vines, constricting autonomy and suffocating confidence. When your reality doesn't match the ideal, guilt and shame can follow, leaving you isolated and self-questioning.

Family expectations compound the pressure. Perhaps your own mother, grandmother, or siblings offered advice rooted in their experiences: "We all did it this way, you'll be fine" or "Just push through the pain." Even if well-intentioned, these statements often dismiss the uniqueness of your body, your baby, and your circumstances. Anthropologically, communal knowledge was historically a lifeline — passed down from experienced caregivers — but it relied on observation and adaptation, not rigid prescription. Modern family advice, filtered through cultural myths, often lacks this nuance.

The emotional impact is profound. Mothers may internalize judgment, thinking, "I'm failing because I can't measure up" or "Others are doing it effortlessly, so why can't I?" This pressure activates the nervous system, creating anxiety, hypervigilance, and even resentment toward those offering "guidance."

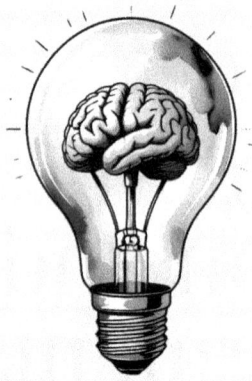

Making Sense Of It
The Weight of Expectation and Silent Judgment

Trauma isn't just physical or emotional; it can be relational, emerging from repeated micro-invalidations by the people closest to you.

Understanding this dynamic is crucial for healing. You are not broken for resisting cultural or familial pressure. You are not selfish for prioritizing your body, your baby, or your mental health. Radical validation — acknowledging that your choices, limits, and feelings are legitimate — helps disentangle self-blame from external expectations. Recognizing how judgment and cultural myths shaped your experience allows you to reclaim your voice, your autonomy, and your right to mother without apology.

Healing comes from seeing clearly what happened, naming the invisible vines of expectation, and giving yourself permission to release them. When you honor your experience without needing approval, you create a space where your choices — even those that diverge from tradition or cultural ideals — are respected. You can finally step out from the weight of everyone else's opinions and recognize that your maternal journey, with all its struggles and triumphs, is entirely valid.

What messages did you receive about breastfeeding from family, culture, religion, or community?

List them — spoken or unspoken. What was "expected"? What was "shameful"? Let it all come out, even if it feels contradictory.

What messages did you receive about breastfeeding from family, culture, religion, or community?

When you struggled or stopped breastfeeding, how did others respond — and what did that feel like in your body?

Did you brace for judgment? Did someone say something that stung? Or worse — say nothing at all? Let your nervous system speak here.

When you struggled or stopped breastfeeding, how did others
respond — and what did that feel like in your body?

What did you wish someone had said to you?

Imagine one person — friend, partner, parent — saying exactly what you needed to hear. Let them speak to you now, through your pen.

What did you wish someone had said to you?

Was there a part of you that wanted to defend yourself? To scream or walk away?

Let that part speak freely now. Give it a voice and the dignity of expression. It doesn't need to be polite.

Was there a part of you that wanted to defend yourself? To scream or walk away?

Did you ever feel like your identity as a "good mother" was on the line?

What did that label mean to you before, and what does it mean to you now? Who gets to define it?

Did you ever feel like your identity as a "good mother" was on the line?

If you could go back, what kind of support — emotionally and practically — would have helped you feel safe and seen?

Let yourself name it all. You're not "needy" — you were simply unheld in a moment of deep need.

If you could go back, what kind of support — emotionally and practically — would have helped you feel safe and seen?

TRACING THE TRUTH

MIRROR REFLECTION

Sometimes seeing yourself — literally on paper — helps separate your truth from the voices of others. This exercise uses a mirror as a visual tool to honor your choices and feelings.

Why it helps:
Drawing and journaling inside the mirror allows you to validate your experience, confront internalized pressure, and strengthen self-compassion.

Inside the mirror, draw or write what you want to see when you truly honor yourself as a mother. This can be words, symbols, or a reflection of your feelings.
Around the outside of the mirror, write the external voices or cultural/family expectations that have pressured you.

Reflect: "Inside this mirror is my truth. Outside are expectations I don't have to carry."

TRACING THE TRUTH

MIRROR REFLECTION

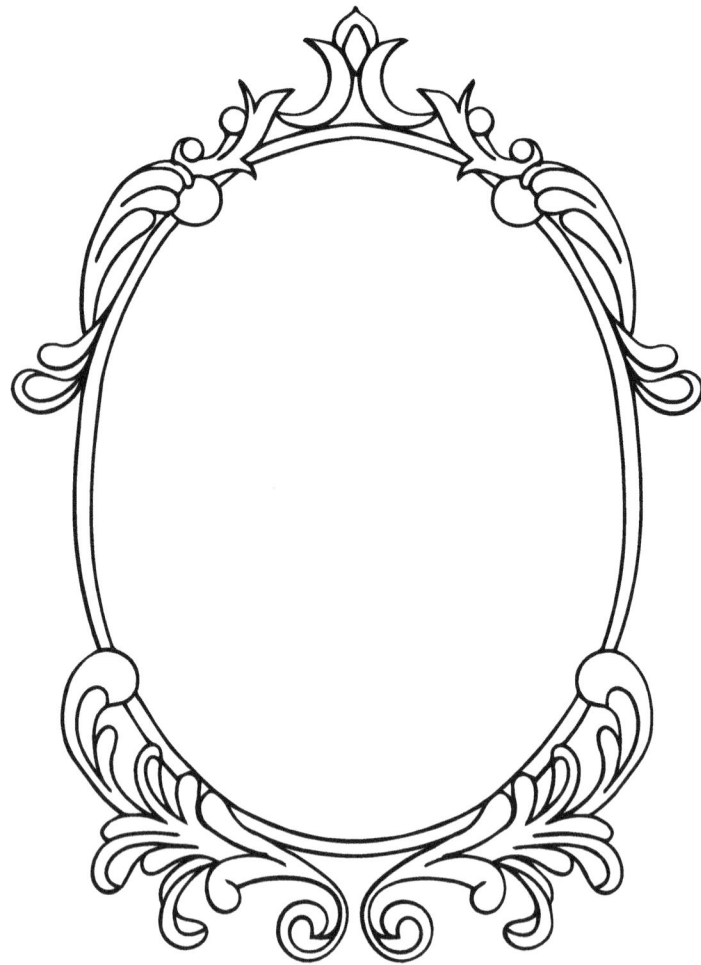

TRACING THE TRUTH

External voices often shape how we feel about our choices, especially around breastfeeding. Naming them can help you separate others' expectations from your own reality.

Why it helps:
This exercise externalizes judgment and helps you reclaim authority over your choices.

List every piece of advice, comment, or judgment you remember receiving about feeding. Include family, friends, strangers, and social media.
Reflect: "These are their expectations, not my truth. I am allowed to make my own choices."

Optional: Highlight voices that were helpful versus harmful, noting how each influenced your emotions.

TRACING THE TRUTH

THE OPINION INVENTORY

Who	What They Said	How It Made Me Feel

BALANCED MIND CHECK-IN

When emotions run high, it's easy to get pulled into extremes—either reacting purely from feelings or overthinking with logic alone. Wise Mind Access helps you pause and bring both sides together: your emotional insight and your reasoned perspective. By visualizing Emotion Mind and Reasonable Mind meeting, you create space for clarity, calm, and grounded decision-making. Writing down the first calm thought that arises captures the guidance of your "middle path," helping you respond intentionally rather than reacting impulsively.

Pause and breathe. Close your eyes and settle your body.
Visualize Emotional Mind and Reasonable Mind. See each as a part of you with its own voice.
Bring them together. Imagine them stepping closer, listening, and blending perspectives.
Ask: "What does my Wise Mind know?" Let the first calm, clear sentence emerge naturally.
Example: "I can honor my feelings while setting a boundary calmly."
Write it down. Keep it as a reference for action or reflection.

Emotional
Mind

Reasonable
Mind

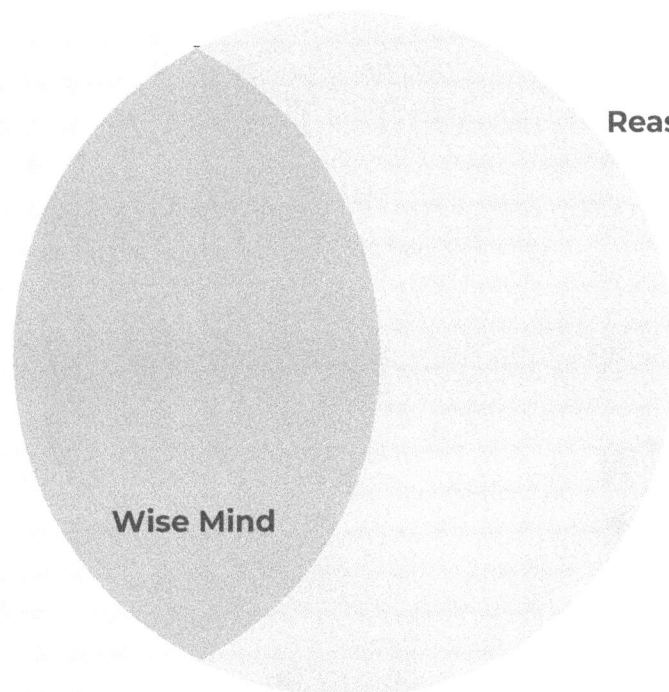

Wise Mind

CRISIS PAUSE

When emotions run high, it's easy to get pulled into extremes—either reacting purely from feelings or overthinking with logic alone. Wise Mind Access helps you pause and bring both sides together: your emotional insight and your reasoned perspective. By visualizing Emotion Mind and Reasonable Mind meeting, you create space for clarity, calm, and grounded decision-making. Writing down the first calm thought that arises captures the guidance of your "middle path," helping you respond intentionally rather than reacting impulsively.

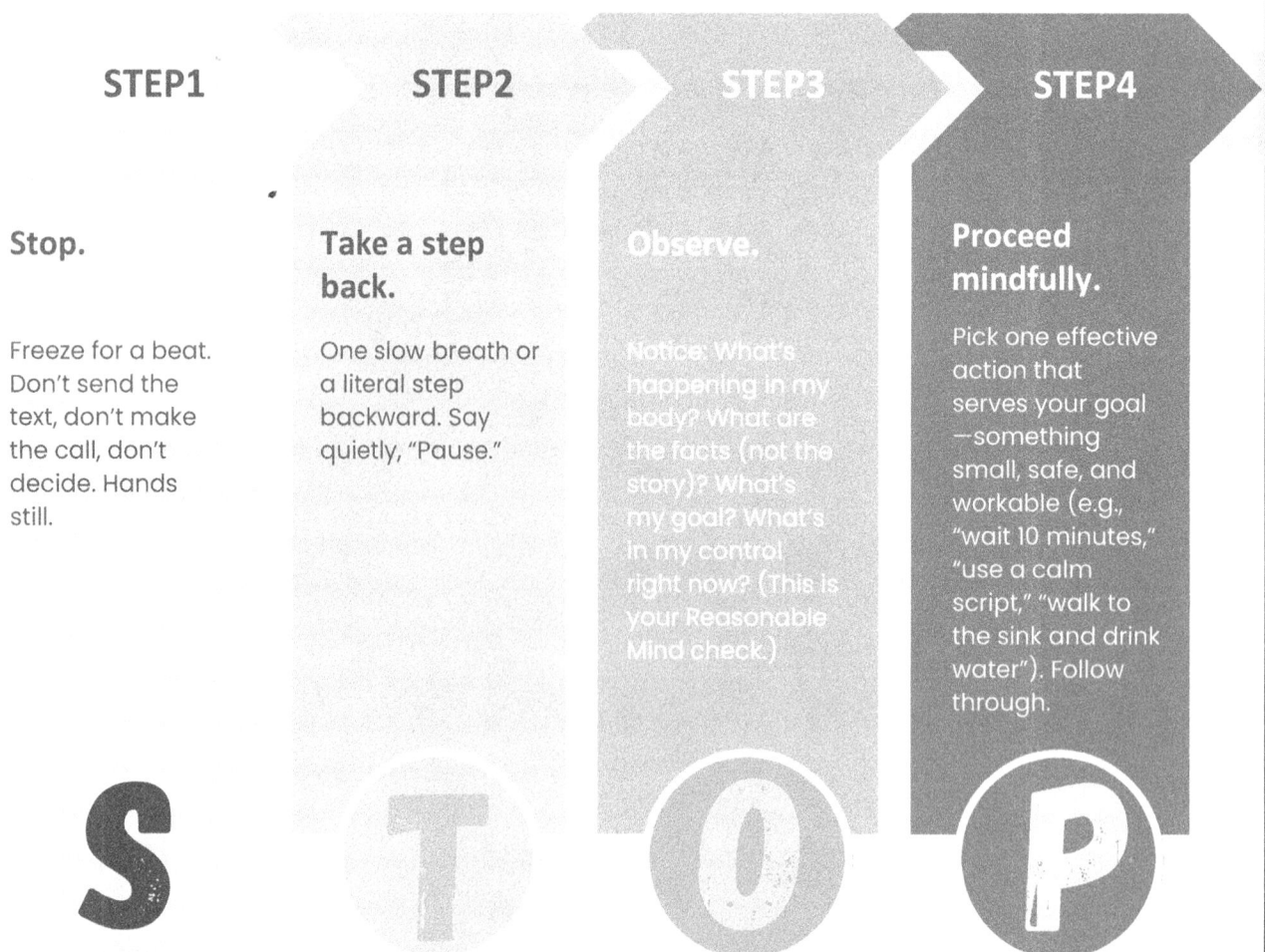

STEP1

Stop.

Freeze for a beat. Don't send the text, don't make the call, don't decide. Hands still.

STEP2

Take a step back.

One slow breath or a literal step backward. Say quietly, "Pause."

STEP3

Observe.

Notice: What's happening in my body? What are the facts (not the story)? What's my goal? What's in my control right now? (This is your Reasonable Mind check.)

STEP4

Proceed mindfully.

Pick one effective action that serves your goal—something small, safe, and workable (e.g., "wait 10 minutes," "use a calm script," "walk to the sink and drink water"). Follow through.

S T O P

SPEAK & STAY STEADY

When emotions run high, it's easy to either go silent or come in too strong. DEAR MAN gives you a clear framework for making requests—or saying no—without guilt or aggression. It balances honesty with effectiveness so you can be heard and respected, even in difficult conversations.

D ### Describe
Briefly state the facts. ("Last week, you didn't follow through on picking up the kids.")

E ### Express
Share how it impacted you. ("I felt really stressed and overwhelmed.")

A ### Assert
Clearly ask for what you need. ("I need you to confirm pick-up times in advance.")

R ### Reinforce
Show the positive outcome. ("That way, we both have more peace of mind.")

M ### Mindful
Stay on point; don't chase distractions or get pulled into side arguments.

A ### Appear confident
Sit up, steady tone, eye contact if possible. Confidence helps your words land.

N ### Negotiate
Be flexible; invite collaboration. ("If that time doesn't work, let's pick another together.")

SECTION SEVEN

When Bonding Breaks — Guilt, Disconnection, and the Fear You've Failed Your Baby

No one tells you how it might feel when the moment you were told would be sacred — feeding your baby — becomes a battlefield. When your milk won't come, or your baby won't latch, or pain hijacks your body, it can feel like you're watching the bond you dreamed of slip through your fingers. You may not have felt flooded with love. You may have felt numb. Angry. Even afraid of your own baby.

That doesn't make you a bad mother — it makes you someone who endured a rupture during one of the most vulnerable moments of your life. This section is here to speak gently to the grief of a bond that didn't begin the way you hoped. Whether you were too exhausted, too overwhelmed, or too hurt to connect in the way you imagined, your story still deserves tenderness. There's still time for love. Bonding isn't a single magical act. It's a relationship — and relationships can heal.

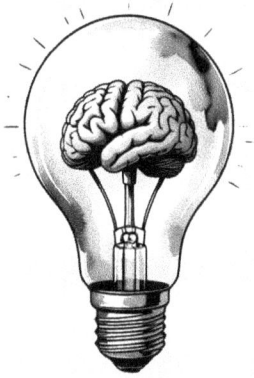

Making Sense Of It
Understanding Bonding Beyond the Myth

Bonding with a baby is often sold to mothers as instantaneous, effortless, and unbreakable — a cinematic moment of eye contact, skin-to-skin warmth, and mutual recognition. In reality, bonding is a process, not a performance. When breastfeeding struggles, exhaustion, pain, or trauma interfere, that idealized narrative becomes a source of shame, guilt, and fear. You may feel like you've failed — but what you're feeling is grief for a connection that hasn't yet unfolded, not a reflection of your love or capability.

Culturally, mothers are told that love is visible in the way a baby is fed, soothed, and held. Anthropological research, however, shows that human attachment forms over time, through repeated presence, responsiveness, and emotional attunement — not through a single feeding session or perfect latch. Even in societies with strong communal support, mothers often experience initial disruptions: exhaustion, trauma, or neonatal complications can delay the natural rhythm of bonding. These disruptions do not erase the potential for connection; they simply shift its timeline.

Physiologically, chronic stress, sleep deprivation, and the trauma of pain or medical interventions can blunt the nervous system's capacity to feel pleasure or attachment. When cortisol and adrenaline are elevated, oxytocin — the "bonding hormone" — cannot flow freely. The body's protective response is normal: it's trying to survive, not fail. Feeling numb, disconnected, or even fearful in those early moments is a biological signal, not a moral failing.

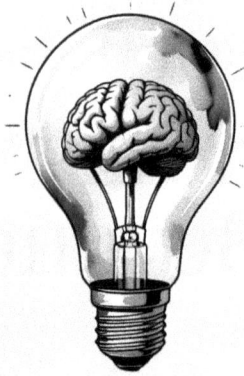

Making Sense Of It
Understanding Bonding Beyond the Myth

Emotionally, mothers may internalize these experiences as personal inadequacy, thinking, "I should feel differently" or "I must love perfectly immediately." But radical validation teaches that grief, anger, fear, and ambivalence are all natural reactions to disrupted expectations. Relationships, even maternal ones, are built over time — through consistency, emotional presence, and gentle attunement. Healing a disrupted bond involves recognizing that connection is not a singular moment, but an ongoing dialogue between you and your baby, where patience, presence, and self-compassion are as critical as touch and feeding.

By acknowledging the rupture — naming it without judgment, grieving what was missed, and observing your own protective responses — you create space for repair. Bonding is not lost; it is simply unfolding on its own imperfect timeline. Understanding this helps disentangle guilt from reality, builds trust in your ability to nurture, and opens the door for love to grow organically. The bond may have been interrupted, but it is never beyond repair.

What did you imagine bonding would feel like — and what was the reality?

Let yourself name both — your hopes and what actually happened. Neither cancels the other out.

What did you imagine bonding would feel like — and what was the reality?

In what moments did you feel furthest from your baby — emotionally or physically?

This may be hard to name, but it's not wrong to speak it. Naming disconnection is the first step toward healing it.

In what moments did you feel furthest from your baby —
emotionally or physically?

What messages (internal or external) made you feel ashamed of struggling to bond?

Did you tell yourself you were broken? Did others comment on how you "should" feel? Give those voices form so you can reclaim your own.

What messages (internal or external) made you feel ashamed of struggling to bond?

Were there small moments of connection that you've overlooked or dismissed?

The touch of a hand, eye contact, soothing a cry. Let's honor the quiet ways love showed up, even when it didn't look like the picture-perfect ideal.

Were there small moments of connection that you've overlooked or dismissed?

What would it feel like to offer yourself the same compassion you'd give your baby if they were hurting?

Describe that tone, that energy. Now imagine turning it inward.

What would it feel like to offer yourself the same compassion you'd give your baby if they were hurting?

Were there small moments of connection that you've overlooked or dismissed?

The touch of a hand, eye contact, soothing a cry. Let's honor the quiet ways love showed up, even when it didn't look like the picture-perfect ideal.

Were there small moments of connection that you've overlooked or dismissed?

TRACING THE TRUTH

Sometimes bonding doesn't start as a single "magical" moment — it begins in fragments. Mapping your feelings helps you honor both the connection you have and the grief for what didn't happen as expected.

Why it helps:
This exercise validates your emotional experience, separates guilt from reality, and allows you to recognize small moments of connection you may have overlooked.

Around your figures, write or sketch moments of connection, no matter how small — eye contact, touch, cooing, shared calm moments.
On the same page, note moments of disconnection or overwhelm — fatigue, pain, fear, or frustration.

Reflect on the next pages: "Both connection and rupture are real. Both are part of our story, and both can heal over time."

TRACING THE TRUTH

MAPPING THE EMOTIONAL BOND

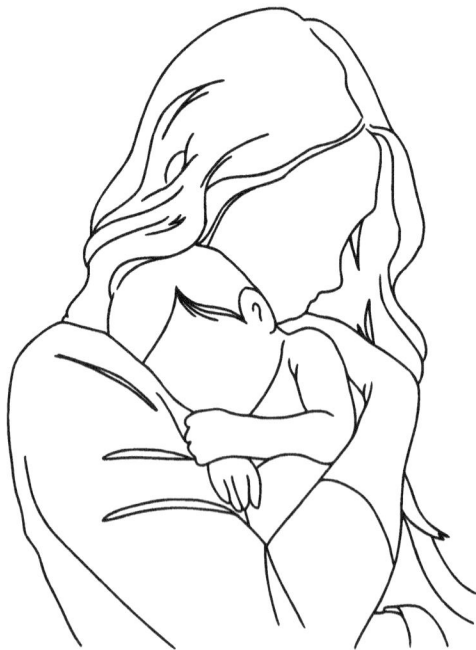

TRACING THE TRUTH

MAPPING THE EMOTIONAL BOND

Reflection:

LONG-TERM LENS

Sometimes we get stuck making decisions because our emotions focus on what feels urgent or painful right now, not on the bigger picture. This exercise helps you slow down and see the real impact of a thought or behavior over time. By comparing short-term costs and benefits with long-term outcomes, you can make choices that honor your future self instead of reacting to the moment. It's about clarity, perspective, and taking actions that support who you want to become.

Short-Term Costs
Example: Anxiety spikes while composing a message

Short-Term Benefits
Example: Momentary relief of venting

Identify the thought or behavior you're considering.

Long-Term Costs
Example: Reinforces reactive habits

Long-Term Benefits
Example: Strengthens ability to pause and respond thoughtfully

THE WORRY SWITCH

Sometimes we get stuck making decisions because our emotions focus on what feels urgent or painful right now, not on the bigger picture. This exercise helps you slow down and see the real impact of a thought or behavior over time. By comparing short-term costs and benefits with long-term outcomes, you can make choices that honor your future self instead of reacting to the moment. It's about clarity, perspective, and taking actions that support who you want to become.

NOTICE THE LOOP

When your mind keeps replaying a worry, label it: "I'm ruminating."

SET A WORRY WINDOW

Give yourself 10 minutes later to think about it fully, so your mind knows it can to come back.

REDIRECT IMMEDIATELY

Engage in a valued action—something meaningful, productive, or grounding.

USE A CUE PHRASE

Quietly say to yourself: "Not now —then." This reinforces the pause and intention.

REPEAT AS NEEDED

Each time the loop starts, remind yourself of the process.

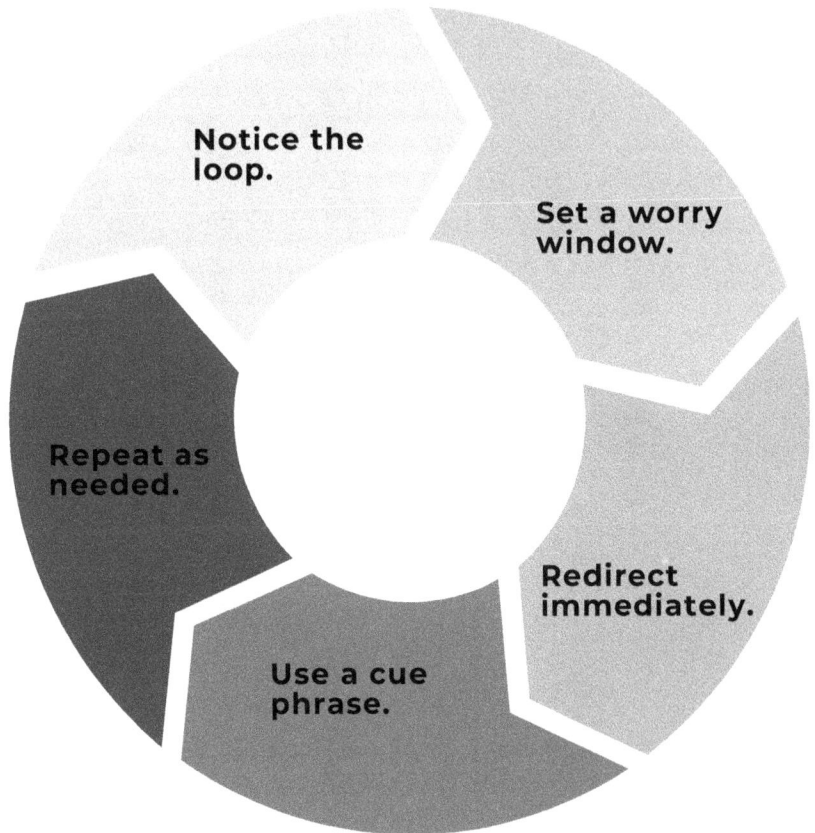

Notice the loop.

Set a worry window.

Repeat as needed.

Redirect immediately.

Use a cue phrase.

NOTES:

....

....

....

....

....

SECTION EIGHT

Reclaiming Your Body — Trust, Presence, and Healing After Feeding Trauma

After months of feeding under pressure, your body may feel foreign, betrayed, or untrustworthy. You may remember the sharp pain, the sleepless nights, the frustration, the guilt — and wonder if your body will ever feel safe or reliable again. This section is here to honor that experience and offer a path toward reconnection.

Rebuilding trust with your body doesn't erase the past, but it allows you to move forward with care, awareness, and compassion. It's about noticing your limits without judgment, feeling your strength without comparison, and listening to your body as a guide rather than an adversary. Through gentle practices, reflection, and acknowledgment of the physical and emotional toll you've carried, you can begin to reclaim agency over your body and your choices.

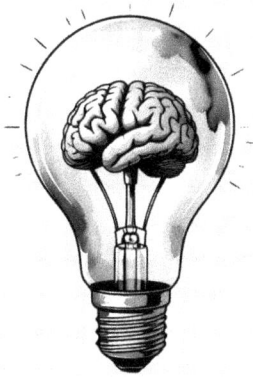

Making Sense Of It

Rebuilding Trust and Connection with Your Body

Feeding trauma leaves a deep imprint — not just emotionally, but physically. After weeks or months of pain, exhaustion, and repeated challenges, it's natural to feel estranged from your own body. You may have felt betrayed when it didn't respond as you hoped, or angry when it resisted feeding, cracked, bled, or became inflamed. These experiences can erode trust, leaving mothers hesitant to rely on their own instincts, decisions, or physical cues. You may catch yourself thinking: "I can't trust my body to do what it needs to do" or "I failed my baby before I even started." These thoughts, while understandable, are reflections of trauma and pressure, not reality.

Anthropologically, human caregiving has always been complex and imperfect. Across cultures and generations, mothers faced enormous physical and social demands — limited help, societal expectations, and the need to improvise to ensure survival. Historically, perfection was never the standard; adaptation, persistence, and resilience were. Today, cultural narratives romanticize seamless bonding and effortless feeding, creating an impossible benchmark that amplifies shame when reality doesn't match. This disconnect between expectation and experience contributes to the internalized mistrust many mothers carry.

Physiologically, trauma, chronic stress, and repeated pain can alter nervous system functioning. Elevated cortisol and adrenaline, coupled with sleep deprivation and constant physical strain, impair the body's natural rhythms and signals.

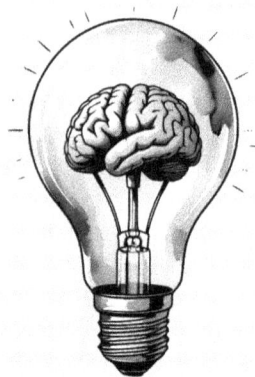

Making Sense Of It
Rebuilding Trust and Connection with Your Body

Your muscles may feel tight or reactive, your joints sore, your chest sensitive or defensive. These responses are survival mechanisms, not flaws. Recognizing them as communication rather than failure is crucial — your body was protecting you in circumstances it could not control.

Emotionally, rebuilding trust is about creating a safe dialogue with yourself. It involves noticing sensations, honoring limits, and practicing self-compassion. Each moment of mindful connection — whether through gentle touch, guided breath, or simply acknowledging pain without judgment — reinforces the body's reliability. Over time, this strengthens the bond between mind and body, helping you respond with presence rather than fear, and care rather than shame.

Trust is not rebuilt overnight. It is layered, patient work. You are learning that your body, though it has carried pain, is capable of responding with resilience, comfort, and care. By observing its signals, listening to its needs, and validating its experience, you reclaim not only your physical agency but your emotional authority as a mother. Your body survived feeding trauma. Your body carried the weight of impossible expectations. And now, it can become your ally once again — a partner in care, connection, and healing.

What physical pain did you experience during feeding — and how did it affect you emotionally?

List every injury or sensation, no matter how "minor" others may have made it seem. Let your body tell its full story without dismissal.

What physical pain did you experience during feeding — and how did it affect you emotionally?

What messages did you receive (internally or externally) about pain being a necessary part of feeding?

Were you told to "suck it up," "it's supposed to hurt," or "you're overreacting"? How did those beliefs shape how you treated your body?

What messages did you receive (internally or externally) about pain being a necessary part of feeding?

_____

_____

_____

_____

_____

_____

_____

_____

_____

_____

_____

_____

_____

_____

_____

_____

Did you override your body's boundaries in order to keep feeding?

Explore any times you pushed through, even when your body was screaming. Let yourself grieve that override.

Did you override your body's boundaries in order to keep feeding?

How does your body feel now when you think about feeding or see someone else breastfeed?

Notice any tension, numbness, heat, tears, or shutdown. These are signals — not signs of failure.

How does your body feel now when you think about feeding or see someone else breastfeed?

What would it mean to shift from punishing your body to honoring her?

Describe the tone, language, and choices that would reflect reverence instead of resentment.

What would it mean to shift from punishing your body to honoring her?

THE TRIGGER MAP

When you react automatically, it often feels like there's no pause between what happens and how you respond. This exercise helps you slow things down and see the chain of events clearly—what triggered the feeling, the thought that popped up, the urge, and what actually happened. Once you can see it all laid out, you can spot the point where you can intervene next time. That small pause is enough to change the outcome, give yourself more control, and break patterns that have been running on autopilot.

Map the chain: Write down each step in order

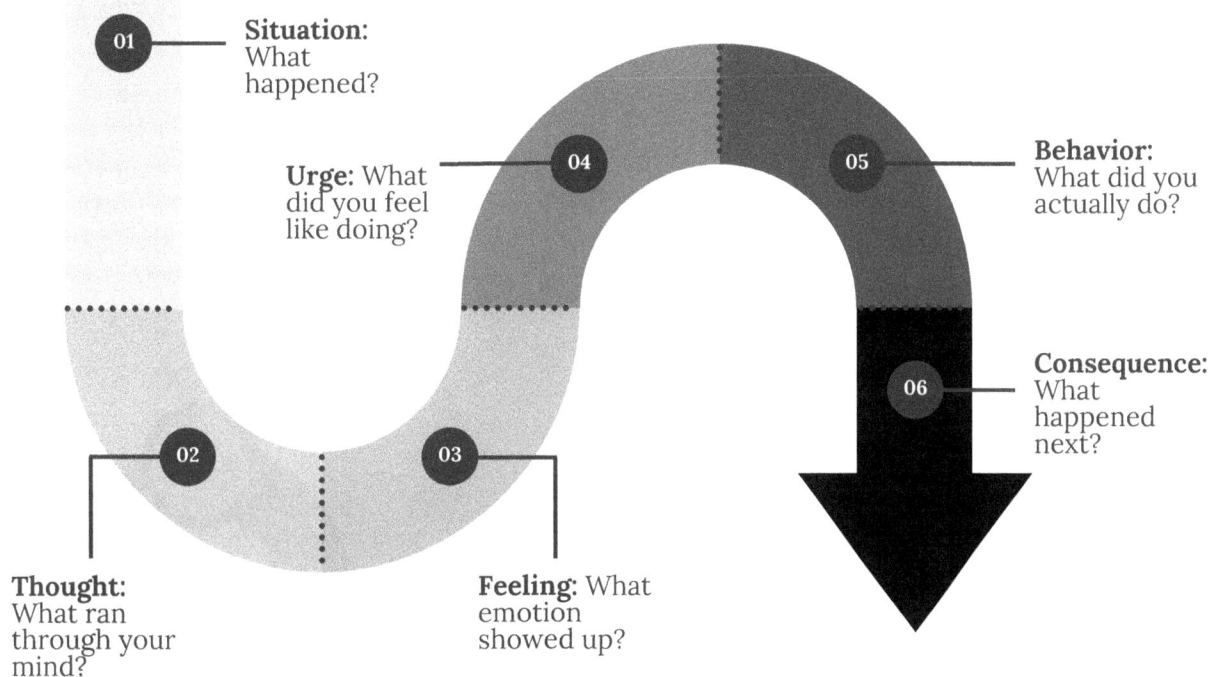

01 · **Situation:** What happened?

04 · **Urge:** What did you feel like doing?

05 · **Behavior:** What did you actually do?

06 · **Consequence:** What happened next?

02 · **Thought:** What ran through your mind?

03 · **Feeling:** What emotion showed up?

Circle your change point. Look at the chain and find the first step where you could intervene next time.

Plan one interruption. Pick a tool or skill to use—like a short breathing exercise, a script you can say, or a grounding move—to pause the chain and respond differently.

MAPPING YOUR RESILIENCE

When life is painful, the spotlight lands on what's broken or lost. But every hard season you've lived through also carries evidence of your resilience. Mapping your past with a "strength lens" helps you reclaim those forgotten skills — endurance, creativity, boundary-setting, persistence, humor, or compassion. Trauma research shows that naming and revisiting these strengths rebuilds self-trust. Instead of seeing your past only as a string of wounds, you begin to recognize the ways you showed up for yourself. Circling three core strengths creates a personal toolkit you can consciously bring forward into your next chapter.

1 **Draw Your Timeline** —Mark a few "hard seasons" you've lived through on the timeline.

2 **Name Strengths** — Under each event, write one or two strengths you used to get through (e.g., courage, asking for help, persistence).

3 **Circle Three** — Look at the whole map. Circle three strengths that feel most alive, relevant, or needed for where you're headed now.

4 **Carry Them Forward** — Write them on a sticky note or card where you'll see them often — reminders that you've done hard things before, and you will again.

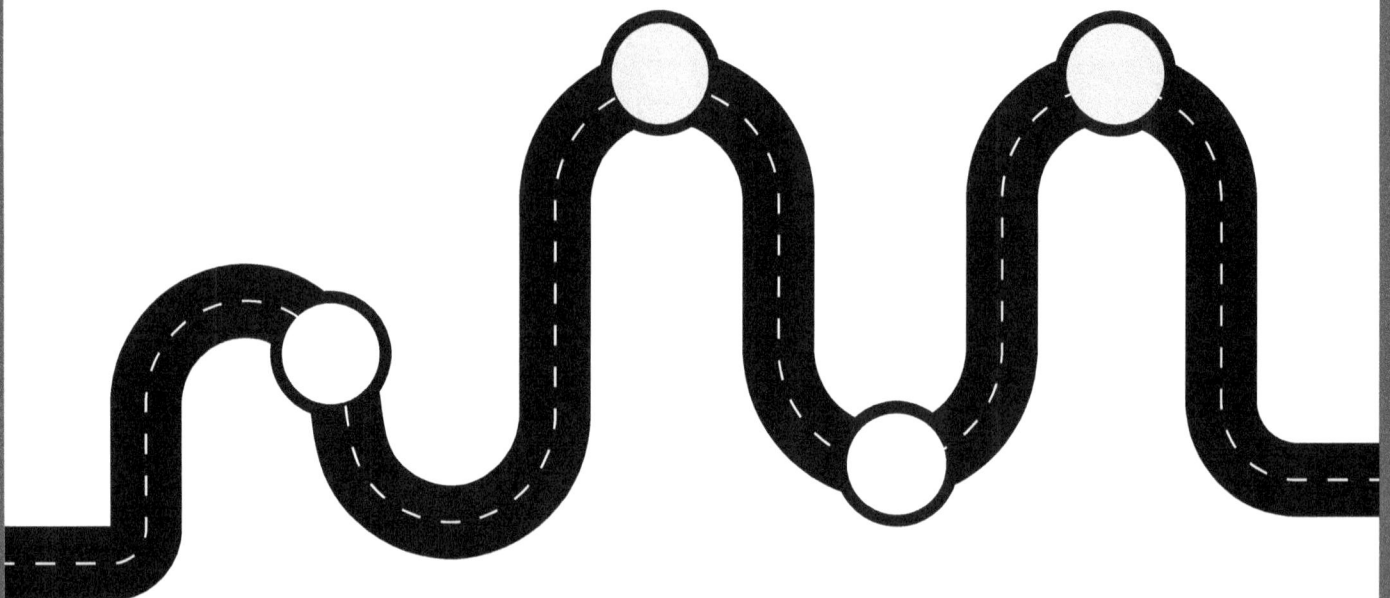

CLIMBING DOWN

When your mind hits you with a brutal thought—like "I always mess up"—it can feel impossible to jump straight to a positive or kind belief. Your brain just won't buy it. This exercise gives you a middle ground. By writing the harsh thought at the top and gradually stepping down to gentler, more realistic versions, you give yourself space to find a statement that actually feels believable. Even if it's not perfect, that 70% believable thought is enough to lower the intensity and guide you toward calmer choices today.

Write the harsh thought at the top rung. (e.g., "I always mess up.")
Step down slowly. Each rung is a slightly softer, more balanced version of the thought.

"I mess up sometimes, but not always."
"Everyone makes mistakes. Mine don't erase the things I do well."
"I can learn from this and try again."

Pick the rung that feels about 70% true. You don't have to land at the bottom. Just stop where it feels believable.
Act from that rung. Let today's choices come from this steadier, more grounded statement.

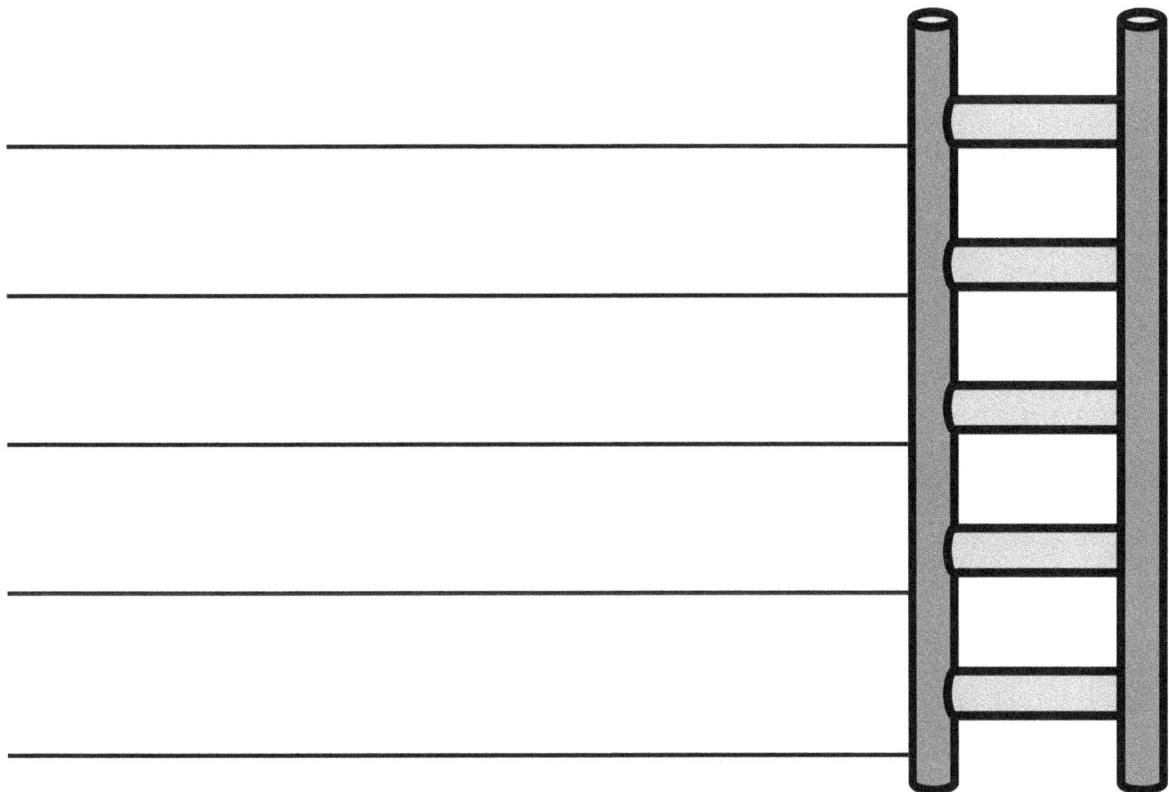

SECTION NINE

The Rage I Wasn't Allowed to Feel – Anger, Judgment, and the Pressure to Be Grateful

There's a particular rage that comes when you're told to be grateful while you're suffering. When your nipples are bleeding, your body is breaking, your baby won't latch — and someone says, "At least you have a healthy child," or "Other moms have it worse." The rage doesn't just stem from the pain. It stems from being silenced in the pain. You may have felt angry at medical providers who didn't listen, at lactation consultants who dismissed you, at the culture that romanticized breastfeeding while ignoring the real risks. Maybe you felt furious at your partner, your family, yourself. Maybe the fury was so big it scared you.

This section is not about getting rid of anger — it's about finally allowing it. Because rage is part of grief. It's part of injustice. And when honored safely, it can be a force for healing. This is your space to name the fire — not to shame it. You don't owe anyone your silence anymore.

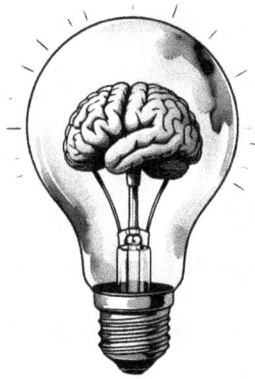

Rage as a Signal, Not a Sin

Anger is one of the most misunderstood emotions in motherhood. From the moment society begins teaching mothers that "love equals sacrifice," a subtle but powerful message is ingrained: anger is unacceptable, especially toward your child, your body, or those tasked with supporting you. When breastfeeding goes wrong — when pain, exhaustion, and systemic failure converge — that anger doesn't disappear; it gets buried. Buried beneath guilt, shame, or the pressure to perform gratitude.

Anthropologically and culturally, mothers have often been expected to endure in silence. Across societies, maternal rage has historically been suppressed, dismissed as hysteria, weakness, or moral failing. Even today, the romanticized image of serene, selfless motherhood reinforces the idea that anger is taboo. When your body bleeds, your milk doesn't flow, or your baby resists, the natural emotional reaction — frustration, fear, fury — is interpreted as inappropriate rather than a valid response to impossible circumstances.

Psychologically, unprocessed anger carries profound consequences. It can manifest as anxiety, depression, numbness, or self-blame. When mothers cannot express rage safely, it often redirects inward: "I shouldn't feel this way; I must be failing." In truth, the intensity of your anger is proportional to the injustice and violation you experienced — whether from the system, the culture, or even your own body. It is not a flaw; it is a signal. A signal that boundaries were crossed, that your needs were ignored, and that your experience demands acknowledgment.

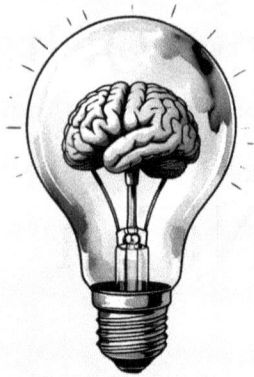

Rage as a Signal, Not a Sin

Anger is intimately tied to grief. It is the shadow of loss — loss of the birth you imagined, the feeding experience you hoped for, the support you needed but didn't receive. When honored safely, rage becomes a compass, guiding you toward what must be set right, what must be released, and where you can reclaim power. Learning to feel it, name it, and channel it without shame restores agency. It transforms what once felt like a destructive force into a tool for validation, self-protection, and healing.

Your rage is a map. It points to your truth. It is your body, your mind, and your heart insisting that you be seen. In this section, you are given permission to let the fire exist — not to explode uncontrollably, but to illuminate, to guide, and to reclaim the parts of yourself that were silenced.

What anger have you swallowed, denied, or judged yourself for during your feeding experience?

Let it be uncensored. This is your place to rage safely, without having to apologize for feeling hurt.

What anger have you swallowed, denied, or judged yourself for during your feeding experience?

Who or what failed to support you, and what would you say to them now if nothing held you back?

Let your truth speak. Write as if the silence has been lifted.

Who or what failed to support you, and what would you say to them
now if nothing held you back?

Have you ever felt angry at your baby
or your own body? How did that make
you feel — and what did you do with
it?

This is a shame-free space. Name it with compassion. You are
not a bad mother for having complex feelings.

Have you ever felt angry at your baby or your own body? How did
that make you feel — and what did you do with it?

Where were you told to be grateful when you were actually grieving?

Unpack the mixed messages you received. Were they helpful, dismissive, or deeply invalidating?

Where were you told to be grateful when you were actually grieving?

What would it feel like to honor your anger instead of suppressing it?

Imagine anger as a truth-teller, not a destroyer. What wisdom might it hold for you?

What would it feel like to honor your anger instead of suppressing
it?

TRACING THE TRUTH

NAMING THE FIRE

Anger needs acknowledgment before it can be released. Naming it transforms diffuse frustration into clarity.

Why it helps:
Labeling specific sources of rage helps separate internalized shame from justified emotional responses.

In column 1: "What Made Me Angry" — list all moments, people, systems, or situations related to your feeding experience that sparked anger. Include microaggressions, dismissive comments, or cultural pressures.
In column 2: "Why I Felt That Way" — beside each item, write a few sentences about your emotional response, focusing on feelings rather than blame.

Take a moment to read both columns aloud to yourself, acknowledging: "Each of these reactions had a reason, and my feelings are valid."

Reflect further in your journal: Are there patterns? Are certain triggers recurring? How has carrying this anger affected you physically or emotionally?

TRACING THE TRUTH

NAMING THE FIRE

What Made Me Angry	Why I Felt That Way

TRACING THE TRUTH

RAGE RELEASE LETTER

Sometimes rage feels unsafe to express aloud. Writing it down allows you to externalize your feelings and process them in a contained, safe way.

Why it helps:
This exercise validates your anger, provides a structured outlet for expression, and reinforces personal boundaries without risking harm to yourself or others.

Start a letter addressed to the person, system, or even your own body that caused harm or dismissal:
Example opening: "Dear [Name/Institution/Body], here is what you did that hurt me..."
Describe specific actions, comments, or cultural pressures that triggered anger, without filtering or minimizing your experience. Include what you felt in your body as well as your mind.
Close the letter with a personal statement of boundary or reclaiming power:
Example: "I acknowledge my anger. I am allowed to feel it. I am reclaiming my voice and my space."

Decide what to do with the letter — you might keep it, seal it, or even destroy it as a symbolic release. Reflect briefly afterward on how the act made you feel.

TRACING THE TRUTH

RAGE RELEASE
LETTER

TRACING THE TRUTH

RAGE RELEASE LETTER

TRACING THE TRUTH

RAGE RELEASE LETTER

HANDS OF HELP

When stress, anxiety, or overwhelm strikes, it can feel like you're facing it alone — even when support exists all around you. This exercise creates a tangible, visual reminder that help is within reach. By assigning a helper to each finger — whether a person, place, practice, phrase, or memory — you make your support system instantly accessible. Glancing at your "hand" reconnects your nervous system with safety and resources, reducing panic, shame, or isolation. It's a small, portable tool that reminds you: you don't have to carry everything alone, and resilience often comes from knowing help exists.

Assign Helpers — Label each finger with a helper:

Person: a trusted friend or family member
Place: somewhere that feels grounding or safe
Practice: a skill or ritual that calms you
Phrase: a mantra, affirmation, or supportive line
Memory: a time you overcame something difficult

Use It — When anxiety, stress, or self-doubt strikes, glance at the hand and notice the supports available to you.

Update — As your support network or resources evolve, refresh the hand with new helpers.

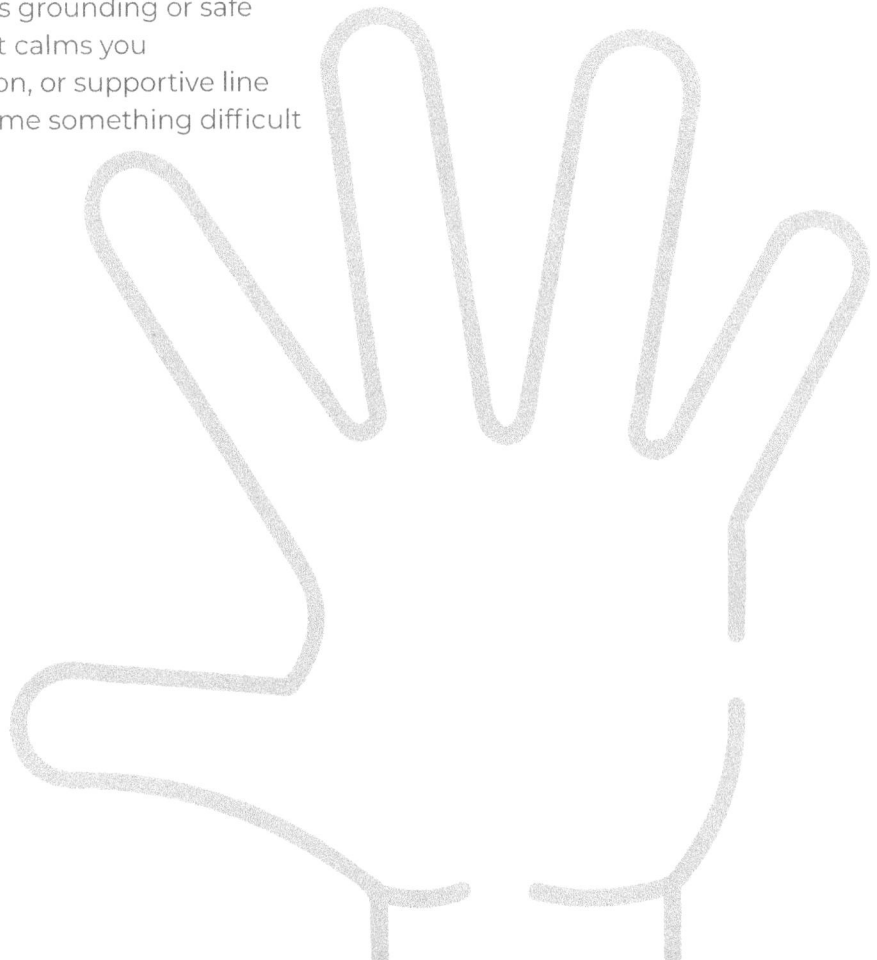

THE CONFIDENCE LADDER

Some moments in life trigger intense fear, anxiety, or discomfort—like standing up for yourself, expressing a difficult emotion, or setting a boundary. When we avoid these moments, the fear grows and feels bigger than it really is. A graded exposure plan helps you face these challenges slowly and safely. By breaking a difficult situation into small, manageable steps, practicing until the intensity eases, and moving up gradually, you build confidence and prove to yourself that you can handle tough moments without being overwhelmed. Over time, the things that once felt impossible feel doable.

Identify a fear or difficult situation. This could be sharing your feelings, saying no, or speaking your truth.

Fill out the 10 step ladder. 0 = completely safe, 10 = maximum fear. Break the situation into small steps that feel increasingly challenging.

Example: 3 = briefly stating a need in your mind, 5 = saying it in a low-stakes moment, 7 = expressing it fully in a more challenging situation.

Start low. Practice the step until the fear noticeably decreases.

Move up one step at a time. No rushing, no pressure—just steady, repeated practice.

Reflect on progress. Each rung is proof that you can handle difficult moments safely, building trust in yourself and your ability to respond calmly.

THE CONFIDENCE LADDER

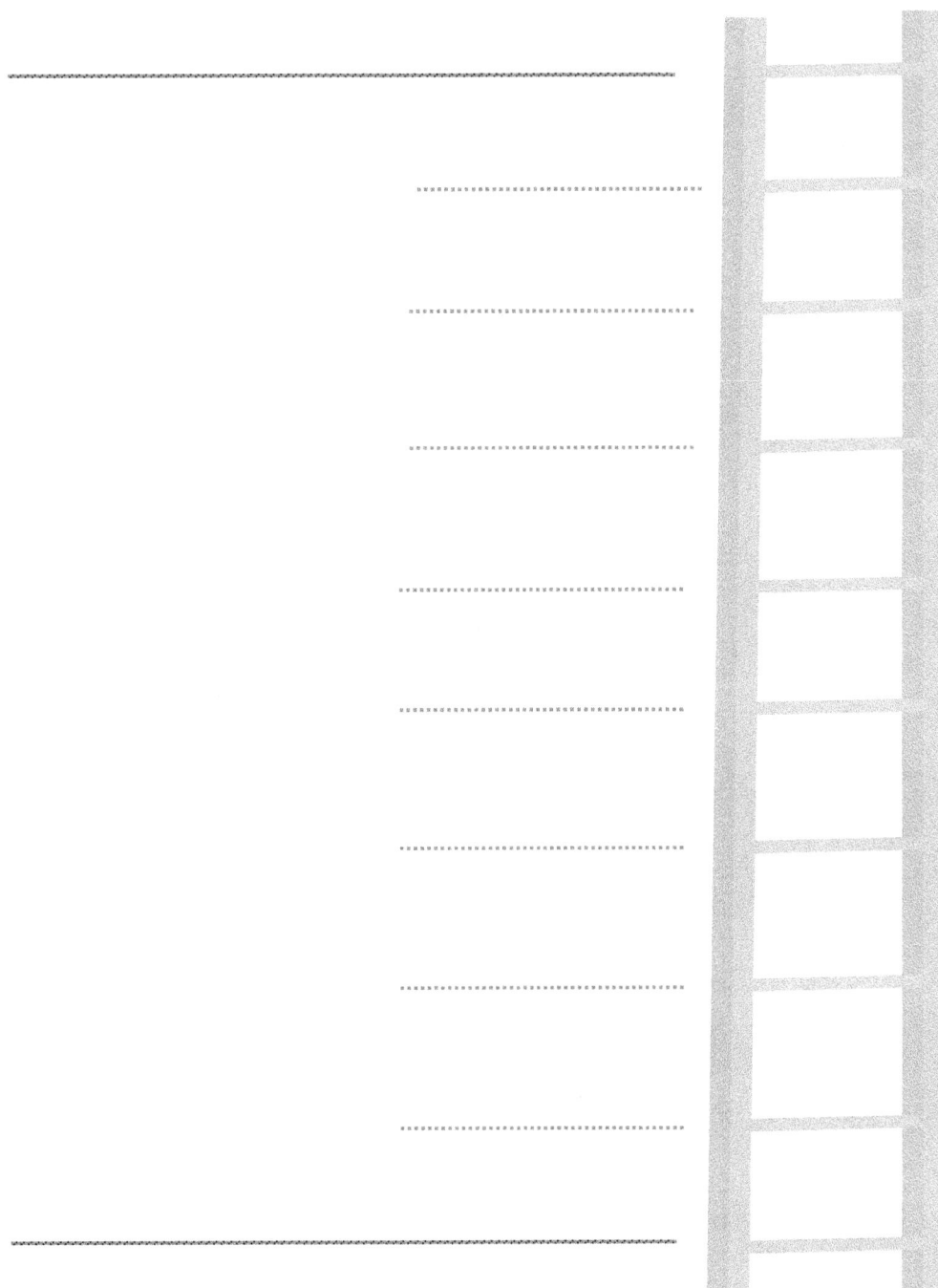

SECTION TEN

It Was Never About Just Milk — Healing the Whole Story

If you're still carrying pain, guilt, or self-doubt, let me say this clearly: it was never just about the milk. It was about what the milk represented — love, connection, sacrifice, worthiness. It was about wanting to give your baby the world and feeling like something invisible got in the way. Maybe it was your body. Maybe it was exhaustion. Maybe it was pressure, silence, or judgment that took you under. You didn't fail.

You loved your baby with every single attempt, every tear, every hour you held on when it hurt. You loved them through your cracked nipples, your sleepless grief, your aching arms, and your silent questions. Even if your feeding journey didn't look how you imagined — your love still counts. Your story still matters. This section is not about closure. It's about integration. About seeing the whole messy, beautiful, heartbreaking truth of what you gave — and finally knowing it was enough.

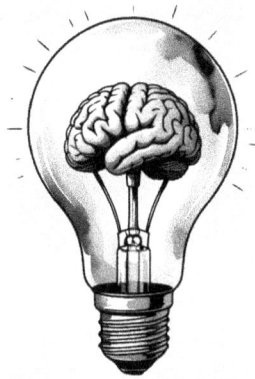

Making Sense Of It
Seeing the Whole Story

For so many mothers, the trauma of breastfeeding is never only about milk. The milk becomes shorthand for love, for connection, for worth. Every feeding — every latch, every drop, every attempt — carries symbolic weight. When it falters, it can feel like a judgment not only on your skills but on your identity as a mother. You may have felt guilt whispering that you weren't enough, shame pressing in because your body didn't comply, grief for the bond you imagined but couldn't reach. And yet, that experience is not a measure of your love or your dedication.

Culturally, mothers are bombarded with the idea that feeding should be effortless, natural, and joyful. Social media, parenting books, and even well-meaning advice frame ease as a standard, leaving little room for struggle. When reality contradicts this narrative — when the body resists, the baby refuses, or the support isn't there — it's easy to internalize failure. And if you add judgmental relatives, partners who don't understand, or healthcare systems that dismissed your questions, the internal pressure becomes nearly unbearable. Anthropologically, across generations and societies, maternal success was never measured by perfect feeding alone. Mothers survived, nurtured, and thrived through improvisation, community, and persistence — not perfection.

Healing the whole story means giving yourself permission to see everything that happened without filtering it through guilt. It's about acknowledging the love, the effort, the heartbreak, and even the rage that existed alongside your devotion. Somatically, your body remembers — the tension in your shoulders, the soreness in your chest, the trembling in your hands.

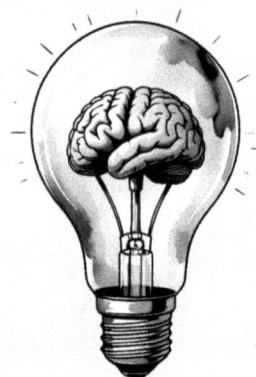

Making Sense Of It
Seeing the Whole Story

Emotionally, your nervous system holds the long nights, the tearful moments, the whispered self-recriminations. Integration requires attention to both: recognizing the physical record of care alongside the emotional record of resilience.

This section invites you to step back and witness the full arc of your journey. Every tear, every aching hour, every attempt — successful or thwarted — is part of a larger narrative of devotion. You did not fail. You were doing the impossible in a culture that asked for everything and offered too little in return. By holding the full story — the effort, the pain, the love, and the sacrifice — you can begin to release judgment, dissolve shame, and reclaim your own authority over your experience.

This is not about closure in the sense of erasing difficulty; it's about integration, recognition, and validation. It's about telling yourself the truth: you loved fiercely, you tried relentlessly, and your care was always enough. The story was never just about milk. It was about your resilience, your courage, your presence, and your unwavering commitment to your child, even in the hardest moments. You carried it all, and now it is time to hold that truth, too.

What did breastfeeding represent to you — emotionally, symbolically, culturally?

Let yourself name the deeper meaning it held for you. Was it connection? Redemption? Worth? Identity? Be gentle with what comes up.

What did breastfeeding represent to you — emotionally,
symbolically, culturally?

Where do you still feel like you need to explain or defend your story?

Who are you trying to justify yourself to — your family? The world? Yourself? What would it feel like to stop needing permission?

Where do you still feel like you need to explain or defend your story?

What parts of you were wounded during this journey — and what do those parts still need to hear?

Imagine each part as a younger self: the part who tried, the part who gave up, the part who's still sad. Write to them with kindness.

What parts of you were wounded during this journey — and what do those parts still need to hear?

How have you continued to love and nourish your child — even if it wasn't through breastfeeding?

List out the real, everyday ways you show up with care. Let this be a moment of honoring.

How have you continued to love and nourish your child — even if it wasn't through breastfeeding?

What would "healing the whole story" look like for you?

Would it mean letting go? Speaking out? Finding rituals of closure? Giving yourself new permission?

What would "healing the whole story" look like for you?

TRACING THE TRUTH

Often, mothers forget to acknowledge the love and persistence they poured into feeding. Writing to yourself helps name it and reclaim your story.

Why it helps:
Externalizing your experience through a compassionate letter validates both struggle and care, integrating emotion and insight.

Begin your letter with: "Dear Me, I see everything you gave…"
Include details about your effort, tears, persistence, and love. Name moments that were hard and moments you kept going despite exhaustion, pain, or doubt.
Close with a statement of self-recognition: "I honor all I did, and I know my love was enough."

Optional: Reread this letter whenever shame or guilt arises to reconnect with your own effort.

TRACING THE TRUTH

LETTER TO YOURSELF —
ACKNOWLEDGING LOVE
AND EFFORT

TRACING THE TRUTH

LETTER TO YOURSELF — ACKNOWLEDGING LOVE AND EFFORT

TRACING THE TRUTH

LETTER TO YOURSELF — ACKNOWLEDGING LOVE AND EFFORT

TRACING THE TRUTH

LETTER TO YOURSELF — ACKNOWLEDGING LOVE AND EFFORT

ASSESSMENT

You've done the work — now let's see where you're at. Take a moment to rate these statements again with honesty and self-compassion. Notice what's shifted, what still feels raw, and what that means for your next steps.

1-10

1 How connected do you feel to your baby during feeding or caregiving moments?

2 How much guilt or self-blame do you carry related to your feeding experience?

3 How comfortable are you acknowledging and expressing anger, frustration, or grief about your feeding journey?

4 How supported do you feel — by medical providers, family, or your community — in your feeding experience?

5 How well do you trust your body and its ability to care for your baby?

6 How able are you to soothe or calm your nervous system when you feel overwhelmed or triggered by feeding challenges?

7 How free do you feel from cultural or familial pressure or judgment regarding your feeding choices?

8 How confident are you in your capacity to heal emotionally from your breastfeeding experience?

Mindset & Identity Shift Reflection

Healing changes the way you see yourself. You might notice you're less
reactive in certain moments, more confident speaking up, or simply softer
with yourself. This page is about spotting those shifts — the ones that show
you're not the same person who started this journey.

In what ways do I see myself differently than when I started?

What beliefs about myself or others are shifting?

How has my sense of hope, strength, or trust evolved?

ACTION PLAN

This is your personalized roadmap for continuing growth beyond this workbook. Use this space to clarify which skills you'll keep practicing, how you'll notice early warning signs, and what concrete steps you'll take to support yourself. Remember, transformation happens one intentional step at a time.

Skills I will keep practicing regularly

Early warning signs or triggers I'll watch for:

When I notice these signs, here's what I will do:

ACTION PLAN

This is your personalized roadmap for continuing growth beyond this workbook. Use this space to clarify which skills you'll keep practicing, how you'll notice early warning signs, and what concrete steps you'll take to support yourself. Remember, transformation happens one intentional step at a time.

Ways I can check in with myself to monitor progress (daily, weekly, monthly):

People or supports I will reach out to if I need encouragement or accountability:

One commitment I'm making to myself right now:

RESOURCE LIST

The resources listed here are shared for informational purposes only. While they provide valuable support and tools for mental health, I am not endorsing or guaranteeing the quality, effectiveness, or availability of their services. It's important to explore these options and verify the details directly on their websites to ensure they align with your personal needs.

National Alliance on Mental Illness

www.nami.org

Offers free mental health education, peer support, and a 24/7 helpline.

Insight Timer

www.insighttimer.com

A free meditation app with thousands of guided meditations, music, and talks on mental well-being

Parenting for Mental Health

www.parentingformentalhealth.com

Offers resources, training, and advice on how parents can support their child's mental health, including guides and printable resources

Crisis Text Line

www.crisistextline.org

Offers free, 24/7 text-based support for mental health crises

7 Cups

www.7cups.com

Offers free, anonymous online chat with trained volunteers, as well as paid therapy with licensed professionals.

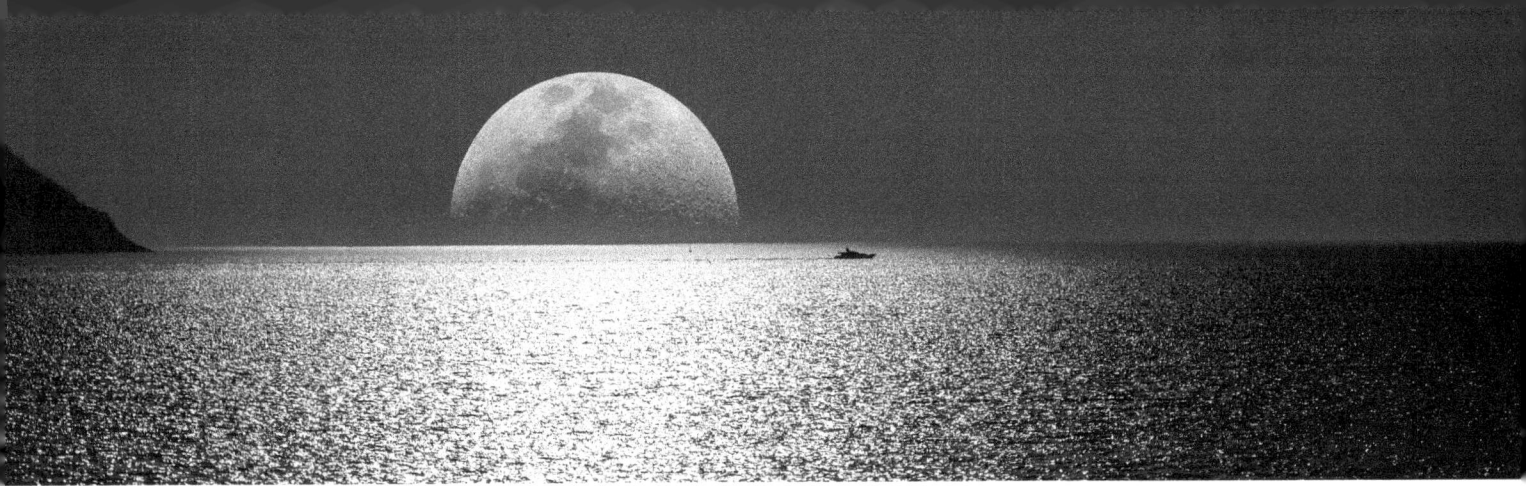

There's a kind of grief that no one prepares you for—the grief of something that was supposed to be "natural" but wasn't. The grief of pushing through pain, through guilt, through exhaustion, and still feeling like it wasn't enough. The grief of all the moments you felt disconnected, defeated, ashamed, or invisible. If breastfeeding hurt you—physically, emotionally, psychologically—you are not alone, and you are not broken. You did not fail. You navigated an impossible situation with impossible expectations placed on your body, your time, your sanity, and your soul. Maybe you wept through pumping sessions. Maybe you lied to the lactation consultant because you couldn't handle one more comment. Maybe you smiled when people said "breast is best" and swallowed the lump in your throat. Maybe no one ever asked how you were doing. Maybe no one noticed you were falling apart. But we see you now. And we're not here to fix you—because there is nothing wrong with you. You were never supposed to suffer to prove you're a good parent. Your worth was never measured in ounces. Your body is not a machine. Your pain is not an inconvenience. You are not less of a parent because breastfeeding didn't go the way you were told it would. You showed up. You stayed. You made decisions in the dark. You protected your baby in the best way you knew how—even when that meant changing course. That is love. That is strength. That is enough.

You are the best person for your baby, even if you don't believe it yet. You always were.

Your love isn't measured in ounces. No one gets to decide what made you a good parent. You don't need to earn your baby's love. You already have it.

M. Tourangeau
Stonewell Healing Press

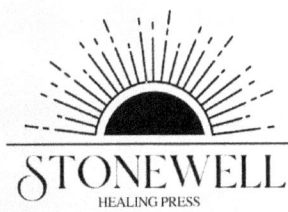

STONEWELL
HEALING PRESS

www.ingramcontent.com/pod-product-compliance
Lightning Source LLC
Chambersburg PA
CBHW080402270326
41927CB00015B/3325